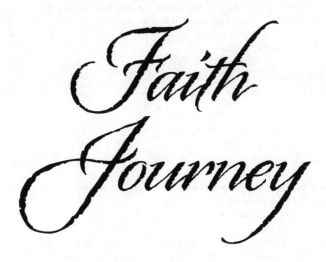

Faith Journey

A Devotional for Christians
Overcoming Cancer

REV. CHERYL TAYLOR

authorHOUSE®

AuthorHouse™
1663 Liberty Drive
Bloomington, IN 47403
www.authorhouse.com
Phone: 1 (800) 839-8640

Published by AuthorHouse 11/26/2019

ISBN: 978-1-7283-3427-1 (sc)
ISBN: 978-1-7283-3425-7 (hc)
ISBN: 978-1-7283-3426-4 (e)

Library of Congress Control Number: 2019917648

Print information available on the last page.

This book is printed on acid-free paper.

Because of the dynamic nature of the Internet, any web addresses or links contained in
this book may have changed since publication and may no longer be valid. The views
expressed in this work are solely those of the author and do not necessarily reflect the views
of the publisher, and the publisher hereby disclaims any responsibility for them.

This Book is Presented to

By

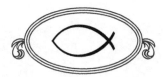

Dedicated to the strongest and most humble woman I know, my dear beloved mother, Dorothy Taylor, who fought the battle with cancer three times. My angel, you have gained your heavenly wings!

May you rest in peace!

Acknowledgements

God never meant for me to go through this alone. There was a community of people who loved and supported me on the journey. I honor and love you!

To My heavenly Father whereby each day He wakes me up to give me another opportunity to get it right. I am so grateful for His mercy and grace! God is certainly enough!

To the entire Taylor, McNeil and Perry clan. I love you so very much. Thank you for dropping everything for me! Family is everything! Taylor Strong George!

To Pastor Jermaine Covington and the entire St. John AME Church family, there really are no words in the English language to express how much I love all of you and how grateful I am for your prayers, support and encouragement! God knew exactly what He was doing when He placed me there.

To my many caregivers, Rev. Dr. Payne, Esther, Dorothea, Fanita, Denise, Tina, Alice, Sally, St. John Women Ministry, Dr. Chidiac, Dr. Vonderembse, Dr. Grant, Alethea, Lisa, Angela, Katrina, Carol, Jamie Lynn, Michelle, Kamaria and everyone associated with the "Food Train"! You all were my ROCK!

To Jan my "call me anytime" friend in support of this book. For everything I didn't know…you knew. Thank You for sharing!

Foreword

I was truly blessed to have a host of family, friends, clergy, church members, doctors and nurses praying for me, taking care of me and encouraging me throughout my journey with cancer. I think of them and I am thankful as I write this devotional. They too were being used by God to fulfill a purpose and to be blessed in their own individual lives by reaching out to me. The world desperately need those who know how to bring joy, encouragement, laughter and help to the lives of those who are in need. They are truly the hands and feet of God.

I truly believe that nothing can happen to me that does not go through God first. This is not to say that God sends bad things my way...it is to say that God sometimes allows things to happen to bring glory to Him, to teach me, to help me to grow through adversity. Remember the blind man? The question was asked in John 9:2 Now as Jesus was passing by, He saw a man blind from birth, and His disciples asked Him, "Rabbi, who sinned, this man or his parents, that he was born blind?" Jesus answered, "Neither this man nor his parents sinned, but this happened so that the works of God would be displayed in him."

Today there are few individuals who do not know someone who has experienced cancer. I know far too many people who have been through this devastating disease. This includes my aunt, cousins, close friends and church members.

I wrote this devotional because there are so many of us that need encouragement and reminders that God is still in control even in the midst of the suffering. He loves and cares about what you are going through. I wrote this book in thankfulness for what God has done for me. He continues to bless me beyond my imagination! This book is for the patient while he/she is going through the journey and even while in remission. This book is also a helpful reminder to caregivers and to others who love someone overcoming cancer.

I can honestly say God's works were displayed in me through this journey. If you allow Him, His works can be displayed in you as you go through your own journey. Nothing you are going through will be in vain.

There is a purpose in your pain, a purpose in your healing, a purpose in the chaos of it all. You will get through this. Cancer does not win. Believe me. You are stronger than you know!

God is truly a healer, full of mercy and grace to those who believe. To God Be the Glory!

Stay Encouraged!

Rev. Cheryl

How to use this Book

- Pray and ask God to give you clarity and peace as you read each scripture and devotional.

- Read the devotional.

- Read the corresponding scripture.

- Go to the bible and read the entire chapter of the referenced scripture.

- Reflect

2 Peter 1:3 (NIV)

His divine power has given us everything we need for a godly life through our knowledge of him who called us by his own glory and goodness.

#Message

I gave you everything you need to deal with this.
-God

1 Thessalonians 1:2-5 (NLT)

2 We always thank God for all of you and pray for you constantly. 3 As we pray to our God and Father about you, we think of your faithful work, your loving deeds, and the enduring hope you have because of our Lord Jesus Christ.4 We know, dear brothers and sisters, that God loves you and has chosen you to be his own people. 5 For when we brought you the Good News, it was not only with words but also with power, for the Holy Spirit gave you full assurance that what we said was true. And you know of our concern for you from the way we lived when we were with you.

Thankfulness

EVEN DURING THIS STAGE OF YOUR life have you stopped for a moment to give thanks? Thanking God for the blessings you have even in the midst of this illness, in the midst of this surgery, in the midst of the treatments. Give Thanks. There is always something to give thanks for. From the small victories to the large ones. Give thanks for what is and what is not. Give thanks for what could have been and what didn't happen.

It is when we give thanks that we begin to find the joy in life. When we are grateful, we remember the blessings of life and not just the trials. Giving thanks is a way of praising and appreciating the God who gave life to you.

Let words of thankfulness flow from your lips and your heart. Watch how your perception of life starts to change and all the blessings you've already received come to mind.

Be Thankful!

Deuteronomy 4:29 (NLT)

But from there you will search again for the Lord your God. And if you search for him with all your heart and soul, you will find him.

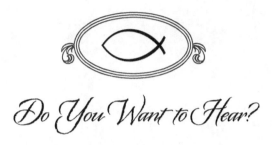

Do You Want to Hear?

THERE ARE TIMES WHEN WE GET so desperate that we don't hear God speaking to us. We become so consumed with our condition that God seems so far away that we may wonder if God is seeing what is going on. The question is not, does God not know, hear and see what is going on but are you now ready to hear from God about what is going on?

It is sometimes interesting to me when people are in trouble that the first person they run to is a parent, friend or spouse, but not God. God is always a secondary resource for them. An "if nothing else works" solution. When questions arise the first source you should run to is God in prayer, asking Him to reveal to you His solutions. That solution will be through individuals or other options. When you go to God in prayer be open to whatever way He responds to you. God does not work on our level of solutions. His miracles are far more advanced than our inventions of resolutions.

You will know that you have heard from God when you have a sense of peace about your situation. Keep your heart open to miracles.

Galatians 6:2 (NLT)

Share each other's burdens, and in this way obey the law of Christ.

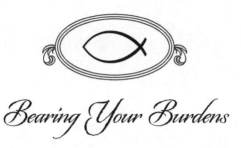

Bearing Your Burdens

ONE OF THE GOOD THINGS ABOUT going through a trial, yes, there can be good things, is knowing that God has commanded others to help you. Galatians 6:2 tells us to bear one another burdens and so fulfill the law of Christ.

Christ has already set others up so they know what they will need to do when others are in need. It is part of being a Christian and it is our duty. Bearing your burdens with you is a way we show love to each other, thus fulfilling the commands of God. Bearing the burdens of others also helps us because we learn to appreciate what we have, we remember not to take anything for granted.

Everyone in this life will go through something. Sooner or later you will have trouble. How you see the situation will either help or hinder the resolution. Whether your faith is the size of a mustard seed or as great as Abraham's it will be the key to the resolution of your trials.

A key to the resolution of your trial is knowing that even if the burden is not removed and strength is given to you to endure, then the strength IS a resolution and it is the blessing you've asked for.

John 13:7 (NLT)

*Jesus replied, "You don't understand now what
I am doing, but someday you will."*

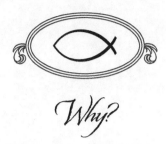

Why?

Why did this happen to me?
Why did this happen now? When everything was going so great?
Why am I being punished?
Why didn't I do a better job of taking care of myself?
Why does my family have to suffer like this?
Why does it cost so much?
Why is my life being interrupted?
Why doesn't God hear my prayers/cry?
Why did I survive and others did not?

ANY OF THESE QUESTIONS SOUND FAMILIAR. The reality is that you will have questions. There will be many questions before it's all over. Some of these questions will be answered in time. Other questions may never be answered. You have to be ok with this. You have to be ok with it because otherwise it will submerge you in to searching for something that is not meant to be found. This is what you do. Change your questions! Speak life into your statements!

This has happened to me...what do I want to do to make the most of my life moving forward?

I'm here and God is on my side.

What promises of God should I speak to and claim as my own right now?

How can I use this situation to bring glory to God?

Who can I contact to help me as I change my lifestyle?

Speak life to your situation and remember that God has the answers to all the questions so trust Him with the answers.

Psalm 25:16 (NLT)

Turn to me and have mercy, for I am alone and in deep distress.

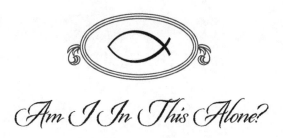

Am I In This Alone?

I KNOW. YOU FEEL SO ALONE. At some point in our lives we will all feel alone. It is usually when we are going through something in our lives. No one could really know what it feels like. They can empathize, they can cry with you, they can encourage you. But you still feel alone.

May I suggest looking beyond human help and company and remember that God is going through this with you. Who knows your body better than your Creator? Every intricate cell was created by him, every vein, every muscle, every cell and every bit of DNA in you. Who better to share your pain and struggle with than the one who wove you together? He is also the one who can put you back together, just like new.

David cried out in Psalm 25:16. He said "Turn to me and be gracious to me, for I am lonely and afflicted." Even David, a warrior, strong, a man after God's own heart felt lonely at times.

Remember that there will be lonely times and times when you feel no one really understands. God sees all and knows all. Allow him to comfort you in your loneliness as you meditate on his word.

Mark 11:24 (NLT)

*I tell you, you can pray for anything, and if you believe
that you've received it, it will be yours.*

Shout Now

THERE IS A GOSPEL SONG WRITTEN by singer and songwriter, Walter Hawkins that I loved to listen to as I was driving in my car. It is entitled "Don't Wait Til The Battle Is Over, Shout Now." While going through my treatments I even wrote a sermon with this title. I enjoyed listening to this song because it was a constant reminder that when all this suffering is over that I was going to be able to look back on all of it and have a tremendous testimony. It reminded me that I can celebrate now because one day I was going to be shouting to the fact that I was healed, restored and made new.

I would be made new because after this experience I would never be the same. My relationships would be different, my perspective would be different and BETTER, my time would be valued more!

My relationships are different because my true friends stepped up and showed that they were my friends beyond what I could do for them but that they were there with me even in the hard times. They showed themselves to be unselfish and sacrificial. They did more than pray, although I needed a lot of that, they did practical things. One of the biggest things I learned about my relationships is that; I needed them! If God thought we would be ok alone, he may have created islands for each person to live alone. God knew that relationships were important from the beginning of time.

My perspective on just about everything is appreciated more including the experiences that I would have with strangers, adventures and trials. We always think we appreciate something the best we can until we come to the realization that we could have almost lost it. Then it becomes a lot clearer and more urgent.

My time would be valued more because I saw people who didn't make it ....they had no more time. But I did. I made it. God gave me more time to do more, love more, teach more, speak more, share more and this is exactly what I'm going to do!

THIS IS WHY I SHOUT NOW.

Matthew 9:28-30 (NLT)

They went right into the house where he was staying, and Jesus asked them, "Do you believe I can make you see?" "Yes, Lord," they told him, "we do." Then he touched their eyes and said, "Because of your faith, it will happen." Then their eyes were opened, and they could see! Jesus sternly warned them, "Don't tell anyone about this."

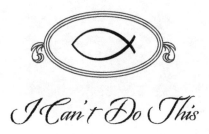

I Can't Do This

YOU MIGHT SAY "I CAN'T DO this." Well, you're right. You can't. That is, you can't do it without God. Sometimes we forget that God actually created us. Every cell in your body, every muscle you move, every brain cell you use. God created it. With that said He knows how to heal you. Heal you to the point that it will be as if you are brand new.

There were times that I would think about the process as a cleansing process. Killing the old cells to regenerate and produce new cells. I am receiving new cells to give me a fresh start. I could start again with starting a better diet to nourish my new internal body.

I think about all the medical terms I learned through the process and I joke about being a "mini doctor." I still become over-whelmed by all of the things I feel I have to do just to get through one day. At times I want to have someone to blame for interrupting my life. I feel like I can't do this. I can't. But God can.

I always knew it, but I had to constantly remind myself that God is in control of the situation. There was never a need for me to feel overwhelmed. I only had to go day by day while trusting Him for my daily strength. He surely gave it to me. Yes, some days were rougher than others but I still saw the next day and the next and with each new day came a new blessing. Sometimes those blessings were hidden in the pain. Think about it. Out of your pain a tremendous testimony can be produced.

No, I can't do it. But God can. He always could.

Revelation 20:10 (NLT)

Then the devil, who had deceived them, was thrown into the fiery lake of burning sulfur, joining the beast and the false prophet. There they will be tormented day and night forever and ever.

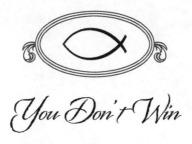

You Don't Win

Satan, here are 21 reasons why you don't win.

1. Jesus is Lord over my life. Not You!
2. I pray and I know the power of prayer
3. I have put on the full armor of God
4. Too many people have prayed on one accord
5. You have proven yourself to be a liar
6. I already have the victory
7. Jesus died and rose again
8. I've seen too many miracles from God
9. God is not a man that He should lie.
10. I believe the word of God and every promise He has given me
11. I will use this trial as my testimony
12. My help comes from the highest power
13. I am a child of the King
14. God has dispatched His angels to surround me and protect me.
15. My God is a healer
16. Your plan for me to doubt God didn't work. This only brought me closer to Him
17. People were saved, encouraged and redeemed by my testimony
18. Jesus has already fought you and won.
19. You were not able to kill, steal or destroy anything in me that truly matters
20. You cannot make me die and curse God.
21. You cannot make me fear death.

Bonus:
I resisted you and you had to flee.

Ephesians 6:13 (NLT)

*Therefore, put on every piece of God's armor so you
will be able to resist the enemy in the time of evil. Then
after the battle you will still be standing firm.*

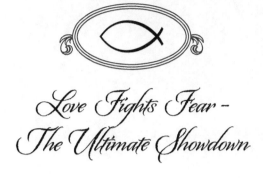

Love Fights Fear –
The Ultimate Showdown

I LIKE MOVIE SCENES WHERE A person is in a situation that seems hopeless, where there seems to be no way out. Then as good writers always do, they create a way out of no way. I like to see the downtrodden win or the victim come out victorious or vindicated. They make for great movies. Usually, at some point in the movie, there will be action where there is good versus evil, the stalked and the stalker, the weak and the strong. There, at that point in time is the ultimate showdown. Someone has to win and someone has to lose. Both are not able to survive in the same space. They are not equal nor or they meant to co-exist. What's always true in these stories is that at some point the heroine is in a sense of panic. The unknown is haunting. The unexpected is scary. Fear takes over and now you react to it. It now controls your every decision, your every move and that fear can be passed on to those around you. In the movie, a voice cries out... "get out of the house" or the darkness is now an enemy as you try to confront the enemy.

In most movies, in the end, the good guy is triumphant. No matter how the movie depicts the triumph the ultimate reason for the victory is that the person overcame the fear. The fear is what made the situation worse. The fear of the unknown caused the anxiety. The fear took over the logic. The fear told you there was no hope. But the Bible teaches us that there is no fear in love. God's love for you is perfect. It is bigger than fear. In fact, His perfect love for you can fight every fear you will have in your journey. But you have to give it to God. Let him know about every fear and then listen. Listen so that you can feel, sense and receive His comfort. The fear will reside, dissipate, disappear. In love, there is no fear. In fear, there is no love.

Love versus Fear. The Ultimate Showdown. Love wins.

1 Corinthians 2:9 (NLT)

That is what the Scriptures mean when they say,
"No eye has seen, no ear has heard, and no mind has imagined
what God has prepared for those who love him."

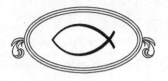

Your Worst Year is Your Best Year

WHEN ONE OF MY CHRISTIAN EMPLOYEES discovered I had cancer she came to me and said she had also been on the journey. She was smiling and with a slight tear in her eye she said "I can't wait to see how God is going to bless you after this. It's going to be huge". I smiled with a tear in my eye and received her words. I needed to hear that. I needed to hear that from someone who knew the journey. Someone who came out of it and knew how God worked. We all know if we are to live life then we will go through some trying times. Cancer is one of the last things anyone would want to go through in life but I Peter 4:12-13 says ***"Beloved, do not be surprised at the fiery ordeal among you, which comes upon you for your testing, as though some strange thing were happening to you; but to the degree that you share the sufferings of Christ, keep on rejoicing, so that also at the revelation of His glory you may rejoice with exultation."***

So now it has been discovered that you have the gene. So now what? A year of suffering? A year of piles of debt. A year of doctors, hospitals, prescriptions, interruptions to life? Yes. All of it and more. But what the scripture teaches us is that we have to remember that power belongs to God and we can face our ordeal.

Yet this year of uncertainty, this year of what you never thought would have or could have happened may have been or is currently the worst year of your life. Let me encourage you with something that I know for sure. I know that in the year of your journey you are being blessed in the midst of your suffering. This year God is preparing you for something greater. In this year you are learning, forgiving, not taking life for granted anymore, praying more, giving up that which took you away from God, being blessed by others who are serving and helping you. God is revealing to you so many things during this time. This can be your best year if you allow God to take the lead and you just follow in whatever direction He takes you.

Jesus' suffering was for our salvation. Your suffering is not in vain. You can look back on this and say there was more good than bad.

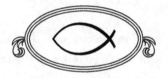

Daniel 8:27 (MSG)

"I, Daniel, walked around in a daze, unwell for days. Then I got a grip on myself and went back to work taking care of the king's affairs. But I continued to be upset by the vision. I couldn't make sense of it."

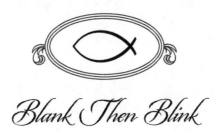

Blank Then Blink

YOU HAVE CANCER. A FEW OF the only words I remember hearing when the doctor came back with the results of my test. It was not until several months later that I was able to breathe, be alone with my thoughts and gaze out the window and with a blank stare just think …Wow! No other words. Just Wow! At that moment I realized I had no words for what I was going through and no thoughts that could truly explain the condition of my heart and mind. Wow! was the only thing I could come up with in my mind.

Then I blinked and realized that I don't have any choice but to go through this. I didn't want to but God allowed it. I had to claim every promise He has given me about never leaving me, every word about His protection, strength and love. When I blinked it helped me remember that God still had a purpose for my life.

Exodus 15:11 (NLT)

"Who is like you among the gods, O Lord— glorious in holiness, awesome in splendor, performing great wonder?"

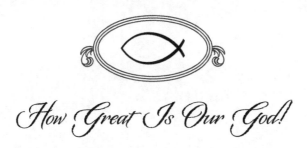

How Great Is Our God!

THAT SONG "How GREAT IS OUR God" keeps illuminating through my head. It won't stop. I don't want it to stop. Our God is a great God. No matter what we are going through or what we are about to face. God knows our every care and every prayer. Our God is so great that He performs miracles right in front of our eyes and the saddest thing is that we sometimes don't even notice it.

In the book of John 9:2, this passage of scripture asks the question to Jesus about the man who was blind. "Master," his disciples asked him, "why was this man born blind? Was it a result of his own sins or those of his parents?" "Neither," Jesus answered. "But to demonstrate the power of God."

How Great our God is indeed! The works of God can and will be displayed in you! Trust that God knows exactly what he is doing.

Job 5:19 (NLT)

From six disasters he will rescue you; even in the seventh, he will keep you from evil.

Simply...Help

Help Lord...

I'm depending on you because I don't know what to do.
There are doctors all over this land and they all need a helping hand.
No complete cure has been found nor has enough people taken a stand.

Help Lord...

I don't understand but I know you have a master plan
I need someone to just hold my hand
I need a miracle right away, Lord I need your help today

Help Lord,

Am I on this journey alone or are you always what I've known?
Can I depend on your mercy, May I have just a touch of your grace?
Lord give me the strength to make it through,
The only one who can heal me is you.

Help Lord.

James 1:2-3 (NLT)

Dear brothers and sisters, when troubles of any kind come your way, consider it an opportunity for great joy. For you know that when your faith is tested, your endurance has a chance to grow.

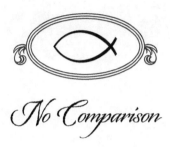

No Comparison

THE PAIN AND SUFFERING YOU FEEL now are only temporary. Yes, temporary. Regardless of what stage of life you are in right now, your condition is temporary. The prognosis is temporary, the treatments are temporary. In Romans 8:18 Paul says "for I consider that the sufferings of this present time are not worth comparing with the glory that is to be revealed to us."

Paul is telling us that everything you are going through is temporary at this present time. There will be a time when all of this will be over. There is something so wonderful that is going to be revealed to you at the right and perfect time. Don't try to rush it, don't try to deny it. If you were to compare it to what you are going through then there is really no comparison. Don't even waste your brain cells. The glory that is going to be revealed to us in God's time will make the sufferings a memory.

There is light at the end of the tunnel no matter what this present situation brings in your life. Trust that God knows and He hears and He cares.

Proverbs 21:31 (NLT)

*The horse is prepared for the day of battle, but
the victory belongs to the Lord.*

What's Next?

I WILL NEVER FORGET ONE OF the reactions I had to my diagnosis. In retrospect, I realized that my faith was being tested. One tear dropped from my eye. The tear was not because I feared death nor the diagnosis of cancer. The tear was because I knew that cancer meant needles. I HATE NEEDLES!

Yes, my faith was being tested and in that single moment I knew God had this in His control. I knew at that instant that everything that God had promised me was still on course and this "thing" was not going to stop my blessings. I knew with every inch of my being that God had a master plan to allow all of this to happen at this time in my life.

The next words out of my mouth were "What do we do next." I knew that God had already dispatched his angels to comfort and protect me with the "next".

Praise God from whom all blessings flow. Can't wait to see what's next!

Genesis 15:6 (NLT)

*And Abram believed the Lord, and the Lord counted
him as righteous because of his faith.*

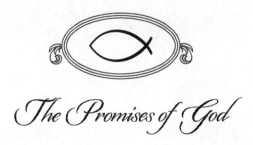

The Promises of God

1. But I will restore you to health and heal your wounds,' declares the Lord, 'because you are called an outcast, Zion for whom no one cares. Jeremiah 30:17

2. For men are not cast off by the Lord forever. Though He brings grief He will show compassion, so great is his unfailing love. For He does not willingly bring affliction or grief to the children of men. Lamentations 3:31-33

3. Wait for the Lord: be strong and take heart and wait for the Lord. Psalm 27:14

4. No, in all these things we are more than conquerors through him who loved us. For I am convinced that neither death nor life, neither angels nor demons, neither the present nor the future, nor any powers, neither height nor depth, nor anything else in all creation, will be able to separate us from the love of God that is in Christ Jesus or Lord. Romans 8:37-39

5. Heal me, O Lord and I will be healed; save me and I will be saved, for you are the one I praise. Jeremiah 17:14

6. I have told you things, so that in me you may have peace. In this world you will have trouble. But take heart! I have overcome the world. John 16:33

7. Whether you turn to the right or to the left, your ears will hear a voice behind you, saying, "This is the way, walk in it." Isaiah 30:21

2 Peter 3:9 (NLT)

The Lord isn't really being slow about his promise, as some people think. No, He is being patient for your sake. He does not want anyone to be destroyed, but wants everyone to repent.

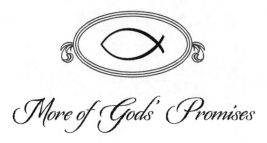

More of Gods' Promises

1. "Have faith in God," Jesus answered. "I tell you the truth, if anyone says to this mountain, Go throw yourself into the sea, and does not doubt in his heart but believes that what he says will happen, it will be done for him." Mark 11:22,23

2. Let us hold unswervingly to the hope we profess, for he who promised is faithful. Hebrews 10:23

3. Is anyone of you sick? He should call the elders of the church to pray over him and anoint him with oil in the name of the Lord. And the prayer offered in faith will make the sick person well; the Lord will raise him up. If he has sinned, he will be forgiven. Therefore, confess your sins to each other and pray for each other so that you may be healed. The prayer of a righteous man is powerful and effective. James 5:14-16

4. For he has not ignored or belittled the suffering of the needy. He has not turned his back on them, but has listened to their cries for help. Psalm 22:24

5. You can go to bed without fear; you will lie down and sleep soundly. Proverbs 3:24

Ecclesiastes 3:1 (NLT)

For everything there is a season, a time for every activity under heaven.

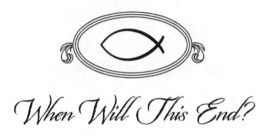

When Will This End?

THERE MAY BE DISAPPOINTMENTS ALONG THE way which may cause you to lose the faith. All I can say is that there is still so much more coming that is worth fighting for. You still have the fight in you. I read somewhere that God gives his hardest battles to His strongest shoulders. That's you. God is not punishing you. He is not playing games with your life. In fact, the reality is that God is using this to show you love. You have to remember that love will show up to you in so many different ways. You will experience love through acts of compassion, empathy, kindness and giving.

The truth of the matter is that you may never be the same again. Your whole perspective on life will change. Maybe that's a good thing. You don't want to forget this. You don't want the lessons to end. Yes, you want the pain to end, the treatments, doctor appointments and everything negative to end. But you'll want the love that is shown to you through the assignments of God to continue. There is so much for you to see when this all ends. Even death, when you are a Christian will bring joy in the end times. Keep your eyes on the prize which is Christ Jesus.

1 Corinthians 2:9 says "But as it is written, eye hath not seen, nor ear heard, neither have entered into the heart of man, the things which God hath prepared for them that love him."

God has something great prepared for you. Hang in there!

1 Samuel 1:10 (NLT)

Hannah was in deep anguish, crying bitterly as she prayed to the Lord.

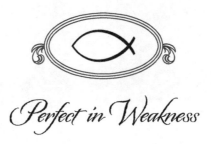

Perfect in Weakness

THROUGHOUT THIS CANCER JOURNEY YOU WILL feel weak. Some spiritually, some physically and even some mentally. Take comfort in knowing that God knows and understands we feel weak on some days. In spite of weaknesses we are still a masterpiece in the eyes of our creator. God has the power to strengthen us internally. Take joy in the fact that Christs' power is made perfect in weakness. It is so important to know that the power and grace of Jesus make all our afflictions livable. You have heard "God will not give us more than we can bear". Allow me to tweak that quote and say God will give us the power to bear our infirmities.

Do you remember a time when you felt healthy, well and strong? Remember the joy you had in life and for life. The joy you had in the Lord? Well, don't forget God is the same God now as He was then. In the bible, Paul says he "all the more gladly boast in my weaknesses." Paul says this because he already knows that God can and will get the glory for his healing and the result is that Christ's power is shown even greater in our weakness. God does not desire for us to be sick but desires to help us understand our need for him and the greatness of his power. We don't have the human strength to overcome our weaknesses. But God does and God can. The grace, mercy and glory of God can be displayed during this time in your life. Allow God to work through you. Be an open vessel willing to let God reveal His power in you. He can do it.

Micah 1:3 (NLT)

Look! The Lord is coming! He leaves his throne in heaven and tramples the heights of the earth.

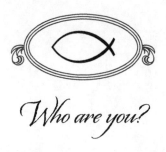

Who are you?

THE SCRIPTURES SAY "WHO ARE WE that God would be mindful of us?" Good question. Who are we? Wow! God thinks we are something great. God thinks we are worth saving. God thinks we are worth healing. God says that He loves us. I believe that, I truly believe that. So the question is asked; why do you have to go through this? Did you do something, did you not do something, did you say something, did you not forgive someone? Did you not do the things you were called by God to do? Were you obedient? Disobedient? Why?

In life things are going to happen. Things always happen. You can be the best person on this earth and things are going to happen to you. Jesus was perfect and things happened to him. I don't believe God enjoys seeing us suffer or in pain. I do believe God uses our pain and situations to heal us spiritually and to allow us to heal from everything that we go through if we let him. He uses forgiveness, grace, mercy and our experiences. He uses all those things to bring us into a closer relationship with Him. It is when we are in a closer relationship that we begin to truly see that everything we are going through is temporary. Everything we suffer is not permanent but is a journey… the journey sometimes is rough but it's worth it. It's worth it if we know that at the end of the day better is coming. That this is not the end but the beginning of something new that God has for us.

It can be spectacular when God starts to reveal His plan and purpose for all of this. One thing I know for sure is that nothing can happen to us without first going through God. I believe he is our protector. God does not bring some things on us but he allows some things. It is part of the journey. I love to think of it as, if God allowed it then he is going to enable me to get through it. He is going to give me whatever I need to get through to the next day; through the tears and the pain. Through the frustration of it all, I know God has a plan. Sometimes God allows us to see the plan in the midst of it. That is what brought me hope.

Galatians 3:28 (NLT)

There is no longer Jew or Gentile, slave or free, male and female. For you are all one in Christ Jesus.

The Secret

ONE FACT ABOUT CANCER IS THAT it does not discriminate. It does not only choose the rich or the poor. Young or the old. The Christian or Non-Christian. It just hits whomever it chooses. This time it chose you. However, let me share a secret with you and ask you this question when battling cancer. From what perspective do you see your diagnosis? Do you see it from the doctors' opinion and expert knowledge? Do you see it from how you feel and what you think? Do you see it from what you heard from someone else who had cancer? Or do you see it from the perspective of the power of God?

The reality is that you can overcome and conquer and still have joy with this diagnosis. Yes, I know the comment "still have joy" is shocking. The secret is that you have to look at this through the perspective of the power and wisdom of God. When you do this everything about how you perceive your situation will change. Your entire approach to each day will be different. Your hope will be more defined and your thoughts will be directed toward the mountain mover and not the mountain.

Several people put their hope and belief in doctors and modern medicine. Put your hope and confidence in God. When your mind wanders and fears start to press into your mind and spirit, turn your thoughts to God's promises. Think about how good He is and has been to you.

Nahum 1:7 (NLT)

The Lord is good, a strong refuge when trouble comes.
He is close to those who trust in him.

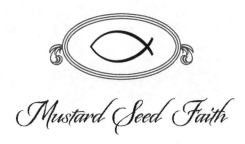

Mustard Seed Faith

YOU MAY HAVE HEARD THE WORDS "Trust God" most of your life. Your Pastor told you, your parents may have reminded you. Your Christian sister or brother says it most of the time. They said it, but not one person told you how to do it. Now you really need to know. You need to know how to trust God. If you ever needed to know, you really need to know now, especially at this point in your life.

I do know that when you learn how to do it, how to let go of the fear and just trust, that your creator knows how this is all going to turn out. That trusting Him was the best way and fastest way to get to what you want; which is Peace!

I do know that trusting Him just takes a small part of you and that's all He requires. The bible says that if you have the faith of a mustard seed you can move mountains. All this really means is that when the power of the Living God is invoked into your situation, into the life of one who has faith then the outcome is miraculous.

In Matthew 17:19 the disciples asked Jesus why they could not drive the demon out. Jesus told them it was because they had so little faith.

Your faith walk begins with your relationship with God. Looking back at all He has already done and trusting and knowing He can do it again. If you can trust a chair that you sit on or a GPS system that navigates and tell you where to go, surely you can trust the one true omnipotent God.

Haggai 2:19 (NLT)

"I am giving you a promise now while the seed is still in the barn. You have not yet harvested your grain, and your grapevines, fig trees, pomegranates, and olive trees have not yet produced their crops. But from this day onward I will bless you."

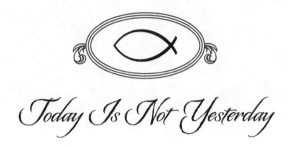

Today Is Not Yesterday

MATTHEW 6:34 SAYS, "THEREFORE DO NOT worry about tomorrow, for tomorrow will worry about itself. Each day has enough trouble of its own."

You are alive today. Today is not yesterday and tomorrow is not today. Love today because you have received a blessing that is worthy of rejoicing. Not everyone got an opportunity to see today. You did. Although today will and has brought trouble and pain of its own. You're still here to fight for life.

What Matthew 6:34 is really telling us is that every day brings something new, something different than yesterday. Therefore, it is worthy of your attention as each day springs forth. The past is gone, the present is your focus and what tomorrow will bring will be in Gods' hands. Deal with what you can today. Conquer today, Be thankful for today. Live life to the fullest today!

When we worry about tomorrow we miss the blessings of today. We are too busy and anxious planning tomorrow which takes away from enjoying the blessings of today. We worry about what is going to happen at the doctors' office tomorrow and forget to enjoy the first sunny day that you've had in a week. Tomorrow will come soon enough but today will never return. You will not be able to turn back the clock and redo what you missed.

Take the time to look out the window at the snow, enjoy the freshly bloomed flowers, sit on the porch and watch the birds look for food.

Yes! The little miracles in life. They are worth enjoying. TODAY!

Amos 3:3 (NLT)

Can two people walk together without agreeing on the direction?

Not for You

2 CORINTHIANS 1:4 STATES "HE COMFORTS us in all our troubles so that we can comfort others. When they are troubled, we will be able to give them the same comfort God has given us." I know this sounds strange but maybe this diagnosis is not completely for you. Have you ever thought about that?

I remember reading this scripture several months after my chemo treatments. I clearly remember the smile and the joy that came to my heart as I claimed this as one of my verses that helped bring clarity to my diagnosis and my entire journey through cancer.

I thought, Wow! There is a purpose for all of this and I'm going to be used to help bring joy and clarity and to help others dealing with this disease. I thanked God for allowing me to be open to His word and allowing it to pierce my spirit.

What a blessing I have been handed. An opportunity to do the work of the Lord even in my suffering. All of this was not in vain. I was not the first person to go through it and I will not be the last. There is someone who needs a word of encouragement and I was to provide it.

What you are going through is not in vain. There is a purpose in all of this pain. Pray for clarity, guidance and allow the Holy Spirit to speak to you. Be open to amazing opportunities that the Spirit will show you. Take this time to grow in your faith and even your witness. You are currently living your testimony. The story is still being written. No one else will be able to tell it or live it. You are blessed with a remarkable opportunity to live a life of faith.

Ruth 3:5 (NLT)

"I will do everything you say," Ruth replied.

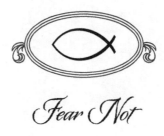

Fear Not

IN THE FIRST BOOK OF JOSHUA God told the people to be "strong and courageous" three times. He also told them to not be afraid and do not be discouraged.

There was a reason that God told them to be strong. God knew that they would come upon situations where there would be a need to have strength. There would be a time when they might have a reason to feel discouraged. Hard times would come and the journey for the Israelites would not be easy. However, God told them to have strength throughout. God would not have told them this if it was not possible to achieve it. With the help of God they could find the strength and the courage to overcome the fear within them.

The God we serve is not a God of fear but a God who will enable us to be overcomers. The fear we may inhabit is nothing when it is in the presence of God. Before this cancer journey you may have had fears. Fear of not enough money, a relationship dying, losing a job, losing a family member or friend. But now the fear may be far greater because it involves your very life. However, fear is a lack of faith, unbelief or doubt that God is who He says He is.

The most important verse in the first chapter of Joshua is verse 5 in which it reads "...the Lord our God will be with you wherever you go". Since God is with you then what is there to fear? The unknown? He knows it. The Future? He designed it. Trust His plan. Fear not. He's with you wherever you go.

1 Peter 3:3-4 (NLT)

Don't be concerned about the outward beauty of fancy hairstyles, expensive jewelry, or beautiful clothes. You should clothe yourselves instead with the beauty that comes from within, the unfading beauty of a gentle and quiet spirit, which is so precious to God.

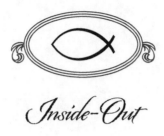

Inside-Out

WHEN I FINALLY VENTURED OUT OF my home after surgery, I always found that many people would say "but you look fine." I may have "looked" fine but inside I was still healing, still recuperating. My mind was still trying to prepare myself for chemo treatments. Inside things were different. The exterior showed that someone cut me and someone changed what was once always a part of me to get rid of something that was no longer good for me. That part didn't show. People only saw the outside. My mindset was different, the way I saw people, things, the future and my destiny, was different. What I was feeling on the inside no one could see or comment on. They only saw the exterior. The shell of what holds my organs, the vessel that I had to use to run this race here on earth is different. Different but healed.

Most people always see the exterior and judge you on that. Not taking into account that there is a spirit, a soul inside of you that needs more care because it is what will last. Care must always be given to the exterior and more importantly, the interior.

Looking fine does not always mean you're doing fine. Cancer changes things. Whether it's your diet, your mindset or your beliefs. Cancer has a way of making people think a lot about life and time. Not that we didn't think about it before but now God has allowed us to look at it from a different angle.

We looked at the world from the outside in. Now we are blessed to look at the world from the inside out. When we do this we are able to appreciate the Creator so much more because we are seeing life through the eyes of the Holy Spirit.

2 Samuel 1:7 (NLT)

*When he turned and saw me, he cried out for me to
come to him. 'How can I help?' I asked him.*

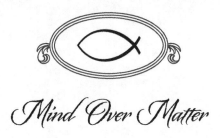

Mind Over Matter

STOP OVERTHINKING EVERYTHING. WORRYING ONLY MAKES you worry more. It is a cycle of neurosis. Only God knows the future. He alone knows the outcome. Even if God has clearly spoken a word to you and divulged the details of the situation then your worrying is not going to change, interrupt or stop the plan of God.

The mind is a powerful source. When it is idle, bad things and thoughts can develop. Therefore, use your mind to develop great and powerful ideas, positive thoughts. Not thoughts to control the universe but to encourage yourself. Job 22:28 says "What you decide on will be done, and light will shine on your ways."

Expect God to take care of what happens tomorrow. It is your responsibility to transform your mind and thoughts to good and perfect thoughts. For this is the will of God.

Jonah 2:2 (NLT)

He said, "I cried out to the Lord in my great trouble, and he answered me. I called to you from the land of the dead, and Lord, you heard me!"

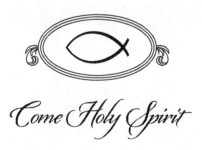

Come Holy Spirit

I OFTEN TELL PEOPLE THAT WHEN you don't know what to pray simply say, Holy Spirit. When you can't find the words just utter, "Holy Spirit. Come, Holy Spirit." Meditate on the meaning of those words. Think about the power of those words. There will not be a time when you call on the Holy Spirit that the Spirit will ignore you. God will always show up when you call on Him. When you utter His name in faith.

When Jesus left, he sent the Holy Spirit for a purpose. He is there to guide you and protect you. He is there to give you the words when you don't have the words to say. Trust the Spirit. He's always there. You just need to call him. We can always trust what and where the Spirit leads us. The Spirit will guide you into wholeness. Mind, body and spirit. It will give you the power to get up every day and fight for life. It is your real source of strength. Calling on the spirit every day you will be reminded that you are not alone in this and never were alone.

1 Kings 8:23 (NLT)

And he prayed, "O Lord, God of Israel, there is no God like you in all of heaven above or on the earth below. You keep your covenant and show unfailing love to all who walk before you in wholehearted devotion."

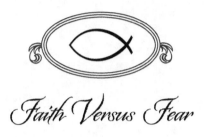

Faith Versus Fear

WHAT IS FAITH AND WHAT IS fear? Fear is not believing, Fear is not being secure, fear is having no hope, fear is "I can't". Fear is "I won't". Faith is God's will. He can do it. Faith is believing. Faith is unwavering. Faith is a strength. Faith is without sight. Faith is hope. Faith is what you need. Without faith you can't please God. It is the substance of things hoped for and the evidence of things not seen. (Hebrews 11:1)

There are too many things in life that we fear however there is no need to fear any man or anything. It was because of faith, not fear that we overcome our trials. Fear is not of God. He did not give us a spirit of fear but of a sound mind. Use what God gave you to get though each day. God will give you enough to get through the day and a fresh supply tomorrow.

Daniel 2:3 (NLT)

He said, "I have had a dream that deeply troubles
me, and I must know what it means."

#Not Even Neighbors

Faith and fear do not belong in the same room together.

Habakkuk 1:2 (NLT)

*How long, O Lord, must I call for help? But you do
not listen! "Violence is everywhere!" I cry,
But you do not come to save.*

Giving Up

You may have a thought in your mind about giving up...whatever "giving up" means to you. That may mean, you are not going to do any more treatments, I'm not going to see the doctor anymore, I'm not going to pray anymore. I will not rest when I need to rest. You're not just giving up now. You are giving up your future. You are giving up what God has prepared for you when you come through this. You are giving up what God is blessing you with right now. It's not time to give up. It's time to push through. You will find that when you push through you not only find something that you didn't know you had but you are giving others permission, the confidence, the hope that they can push through also. What you are going through is also so that the Lord will be glorified. When <u>GOD</u> is glorified incredible things happen. Miracles start to come through. People are restored and renewed and given hope because you didn't give up.

You are here for a purpose. Nowhere in the Bible will you find that your life will be trouble-free. I do find in the bible that God wants only what is good for you. Jeremiah 29:11 says that "For I know the plans I have for you," declares the Lord, "Plans to prosper you and not to harm you, plans to give you hope and a future".

God is going to live up to His promise to you. If He said it. He is going to do it.

He said it so that you can believe it. He said it so that you can have hope. He said it so that you would not give up.

Zephaniah 3:9 (NLT)

"Then I will purify the speech of all people, so that everyone can worship the Lord together.

Help Is A Prayer

How many times will you pray while you are going through this? What words must you find to speak to God to ask for what you need? Sometimes the words, help Lord, are the only words that will suffice. Help Me Lord is the only feeling that sums up everything you are going through right now. The reason Help Me can be, should be and is your only prayer at times is because it is two of the most powerful words you can ever whisper.

The words "Help Me" mean so much more than just a request. Help me means I need your strength because my strength is not sufficient for this task. It means something is wrong and I don't know how to fix it. It is understood to mean I choose You, the Father, to come to my rescue. Help me is a conscious decision to do something about your situation instead of standing still and giving in.

Praying "Help Me" is not a prayer of the weak but a prayer of the one who has faith. A prayer of belief seeks the all-powerful God who can solve any problem. Heal any ailment, restore any loss and do it all at the perfect time.

Help me Lord is a great prayer.

Psalm 94:19 (NRSV)

When the cares of my heart are many, your consolations cheer my soul.

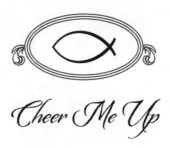

Cheer Me Up

HAVE YOU EVER DONE ANYTHING OR said something just to cheer someone up? Maybe it was an old memory or words that you know would make a person laugh. We do it to momentarily allow that person to take their mind off of their worries. You know it may not change the situation but a moment of joy or seconds of laughter is better than constant pain, anger and heartache.

There are so many studies about what laughter can do for the soul and body. When we are happy, smiling and find joy in the small things in life it brings much comfort to the soul. Many find comfort when those around you are consoling you during times you have grieved for a loved one.

It is the same as our God. When He consoles us He allows us to remember the times He has rescued us from past problems. He consoles us with the promises from His word. He continues to console us when He delivers on those promises. Because the Lord cares about us He continually monitors our soul to help wherever it is needed.

Prov. 16:33

We make our own decisions but the Lord determines what happens.

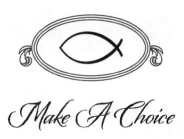

Make A Choice

ONE THING THAT GOD HAS GIVEN us is free will. We have free will to choose to love and obey Him and free will to make decisions based on our own judgement and education on the situation; with or without consulting God. However, the word says that we can make our own decisions but the Lord determines what happens.

This does not mean it is useless for us to have brains and make decisions in life. It means that as a child of God we have the confidence in knowing that even if we make wrong choices that God will and can step in to determine the outcome. Some decisions we make will cause negative consequences. God will allow us to learn and grow from those consequences. Because of God's mercy and His plans for our lives He will also protect us from some negative consequences.

It also means that no matter what the doctor says, only God knows the final outcome. It is only our job to trust God, use the wisdom, tools and gifts he has given us to make decisions during this time and then watch him do what he does best. Make A Way.

2 Kings 5:10 (NLT)

But Elisha sent a messenger out to him with this message: "Go and wash yourself seven times in the Jordan River. Then your skin will be restored, and you will be healed of your leprosy."

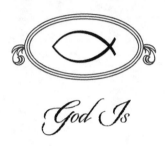

God Is

GOD IS OMNIPRESENT MEANS GOD IS with you in the operating room, the treatment room, the clinic, the pharmacy, the waiting room, the hospital room, the emergency room, the car drive to and from, the visits, the checkup, the hospice room, the elevator and anywhere else you may be.

God is Omnipotent means he has the power to heal you, the power to turn the results around, power to astound the doctors, power to ease the pain, power to give you strength, power to lift you, power to enable you, power to sustain you and the power to deliver you.

God is omniscient means he knows the end to this story just like He knew your beginning. He knows who should be in the room with you and who should not. He knows who should help you during this journey and who should stay away. He knows what you don't know.

God is Omnipresent, Omnipotent, Omniscient and always will be.

Romans 12:4-5 (NIV)

For just as each of us has one body with many members, and these members do not all have the same function, so in Christ we, though many, form one body, and each member belongs to all the others.

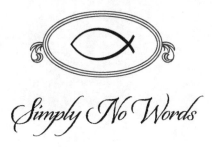

Simply No Words

PEOPLE YOU KNOW AND PEOPLE YOU don't know will have a lot of different reactions to your diagnosis. There will be individuals who will be shocked, saddened, hopeful, hopeless and some may even have a cavalier attitude about your situation. Some will reach out to you others may avoid you. Some will simply have no words. Their responses will not be just related to you but related to them. They will react based on several different criteria. They may react a certain way based on their relationship with you, based on a history with a loved one with cancer or maybe even their personal experience. Some may react out of their guilt of how they feel about you, others react on and out of obedience to God. Whatever their reaction remember they are also affected by your diagnosis.

Well, how can that be?

As a family member in Christ, Romans 12:4-5 states "For just as each of us has one body with many members, and these members do not all have the same function, so in Christ we, though many, form one body, and each member belongs to all the others".

As a member of the body of Christ what affects you, affects me. We all have different functions in the body but we cannot accomplish everything we need to unless other parts of the body are helping us.

Just as a leg cannot function properly without the knee or even the foot without the leg being attached. As a family, we need to be attached in order for us to walk this path called life. It is such a lonely road to travel when you travel it alone. You need people and people need you. Let them in. They are part of your body.

Joel 2:7 (NLT)

The attackers march like warriors and scale city walls like soldiers. Straight forward they march, never breaking rank.

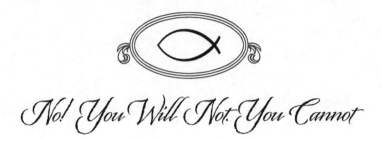

No! You Will Not. You Cannot

No Cancer,

You will not take away the faith that I have in God and His mercy.

You will not make me believe that you have power over me.

You will not make me live every day in fear and worry.

You will not amputate my dreams for my life.

You will not decide whether I live or die. Only God does that.

No Cancer,

You cannot suggest that I asked for this or I deserved this.

You cannot convince me that God wants me to suffer.

You cannot ask me to give up.

You cannot reroute my destiny and purpose.

No Cancer,

You do not have the power. I do. God does.

Jeremiah 20:14-15 (KJV)

Cursed be the day wherein I was born: let not the day wherein my mother bare me be blessed. Cursed be the man who brought tidings to my father, saying, A man child is born unto thee; making him very glad.

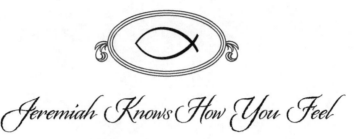

Jeremiah Knows How You Feel

JEREMIAH IS WIDELY KNOWN AS THE Weeping Prophet. Jeremiah was just doing his job and warning God's people of the judgment that was to come and what they should do. What awaited him was condemnation, threats, ridicule and even imprisonment.

You may be thinking that your faithfulness to God and His calling on your life has left you in this very vulnerable place. This leaves you in a place that you believe you have a right to complain. After all, you have done what God has asked you to do. You have been faithful in giving, obedient in forgiveness, consistent in love and diligent in worship.

Jeremiah complained also. When he was done with his complaints to God he remained faithful to God and obedient to what God asked him to do and to be.

Ask the Holy Spirit to help you to remain in right fellowship with God and help you through your feelings of anger and the pressures of life. No matter what the outcome...God is still God and He still listens to our complaints and heals our hearts.

2 Corinthians 1:5 (NLT)

*For the more we suffer for Christ, the more God will
shower us with his comfort through Christ.*

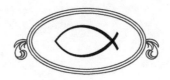

Feelings...Nothing More Than Feelings

ROMANS 8:35-39 STATES, WHO SHALL SEPARATE us from the love of Christ? Shall trouble or hardship or persecution or famine or nakedness or danger or sword? As it is written: "For your sake we face death all day long; we are considered as sheep to be slaughtered." No, in all these things we are more than conquerors through him who loved us. For I am convinced that neither death nor life, neither angels nor demons, neither the present nor the future, nor any powers, neither height nor depth, nor anything else in all creation, will be able to separate us from the love of God that is in Christ Jesus our LORD.

Some people believe that if you are a Christian that you will not experience fear or shock in your life. The truth is that you are human and you have human emotions. Fear and shock is a human emotion. Paul had a feeling of fear when ministering to the Corinthians yet he still maintained his faith. Feeling afraid and shocked does not make you less of a Christian it makes you human. Knowing and trusting that God will give you peace IN THE MIDST of that fear and shock is a witness to your belief in Christ.

Nothing! Absolutely Nothing - can separate you from the intense degree of God's love for you and how much he cares for you. The sin you have committed, the hurt you've caused in the past, the thoughts you have or even the words you speak does not cause God to love you more or less. He died for you. Even though He knew you did all of that stuff it did not stop him from sacrificing himself for you.

This cancer journey is not a punishment or a payback. It is a crisis that you are encountering. Everyone has their own type of crisis. This is yours. With God you can still have peace and be assured that God still loves you and will not leave you because nothing can separate you from His love.

Psalm 77:11 (NIV)

*I will remember the deeds of the Lord; yes, I will
remember your miracles of long ago.*

I Remember When...

When your enemies surrounded you, God showed you favor.

When they said you couldn't do it, you did it and knew God was on your side.

When the pain would not stop....God's grace was sufficient.

When you didn't have the money...the bills were still paid.

When you were weak in spirit......God gave you the strength to make it one more day.

When you were lonely... the phone rang and you were reminded you were loved.

When the pain of the death of a loved one overtakes you...You are reminded that they knew and accepted Christ.

When the job, the kids, the husband, the family, the friends, the relationships, the bills, the church, the debt, the money was not right... God made it all worthwhile.

When God woke you up this morning and reminded you that you had a purpose for being here on earth.

When God reminded you that you were unique.

When the words "God Help Me" was all God needed to hear to come and rescue you!

2 Timothy 3:16 (NIV)

*All scripture is inspired by God and is useful for teaching, for reproof,
for correction, and for training in righteousness so everyone who
belongs to God may be proficient, equipped for every good work.*

Consider This

Consider this: Fact: God Loves you!!! There is nothing you can say, nothing you can do or think to change that.
Proof: *Romans 8:38-39 For I am convinced that neither death nor life, nor angels, nor rulers, nor things to come, nor powers, nor height, nor depth, nor anything else in all creation, will be able to separate us from the love of God in Christ Jesus our Lord. (NRSV)*

Consider this: Fact: God will help you fight your battles
Proof: *I Chronicles 5:20 ...for they cried to God in battle, and he granted their entreaty because they trusted in Him. (NRSV)*

Consider this: Fact: People look at how well you dress. Judge you by your designer clothes and the latest hairstyles. God looks at your heart not your appearance.
Proof: *1 Samuel 16:7 Do not look on his appearance or on the height of his stature, for I have rejected him; for the Lord does not see as mortals see; they look on the outward appearance, but the Lord looks on the heart. (NRSV)*

Consider this: Fact: God wants only the best for you.
Proof: *Jeremiah 29:11 For I know the plans I have for you, says the Lord, plans for your welfare and not for harm, to give you a future with hope. (NRSV)*

Consider this: Fact: You can have peace right now if you listen to God.
Proof: *Proverbs 1:33 but those who listen to me will be secure and will live at ease, without dread of disaster. (NRSV)*

Consider this: Fact: There is only one thing you need to do to be saved.
Proof: *Romans 10:9 If you confess with your lips that Jesus is Lord and believe in your heart that God raised him from the dead, you will be saved. (NRSV)*

Romans 8:28 (NIV)

We know that all things work together for good for those who love God, who are called according to His purpose."

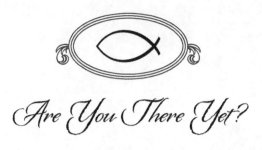

Are You There Yet?

ARE WE THERE YET? I CAN still hear these words from the sweet voices of my seven year old nephew Antwan and my 10 year old niece Jamie. I was driving them to visit the Columbus Zoo. They were in Columbus to visit me for the summer and I wanted them to have this unforgettable experience with Auntie Cheryl. I never thought the Zoo was far from where I lived at the time and viewed it as a short drive but to my niece and nephew, it seemed as if we were driving for hours and would never get there. The excitement and anticipation of their first visit to the Columbus Zoo was just unbearable to them!

We often ask God "Are we there Yet?" We ask him in different ways but nonetheless the same question. God, when is this pain going to end? God, when are my finances going to be turned around? God, when will I see a light at the end of this tunnel? God, are we there yet? God hears your cry and YES he knows exactly when you'll get there.

While you're waiting to get there have you thought about exactly why you're still waiting? It could be that you're not properly prepared to receive what is waiting for you once you get "there". It may be that you ARE ready to receive whatever awaits you but the timing is not right on the other end. Stop trying to rush your life and your dreams. You are exactly where God wants you to be at this point. If you have truly given your life, future and decisions over to God, trust His timing and don't second guess God or try to help Him out with your ideas on how things should progress. God only wants the best for his children and will set things up so that they will have the best in all situations.

Think about where you are in terms of Gods' will for your life. Are you there in terms of being obedient to his Word? Are you there in total dedication to your prayer life, your time, talents and tithe to the church? Are you where YOU should be according to where and what God has told you to do?

Jeremiah 29:11(NIV)

"For I know the plans I have for you, declares the Lord, plans to prosper you and not to harm you, plans to give you hope and a future."

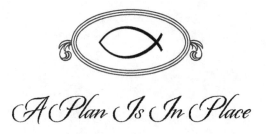

A Plan Is In Place

SINCE GOD ALREADY HAS A PLAN to prosper you and give you a future don't you think he is also going to prepare us to receive it so that we don't screw it up once we get our hands on this wonderful plan He has for our lives? This may just be your time of preparation. Trust God with your future and the timing. You may not be able to see it right now but stand by faith and you won't be disappointed.

Matthew 6:34 (NLT)

*"So don't worry about tomorrow, for tomorrow will bring
its own worries. Today's trouble is enough for today.*

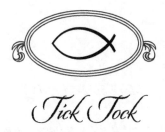

Tick Tock

GOD GIVES YOU YOUR LIFE MINUTE by minute and hour by hour. Remember this when you have a tendency to worry about what is going to happen tomorrow. Only God knows. Happiness is found in the minute that you are living in the miracles around you. You have the power to choose to live happy, to live defeated or to live fearfully.

We all have the same ending. Death. It is the choices we make in those minutes that make the difference. Those choices in those minutes define our legacy. Those hours write our eulogy. Don't take those minutes and those hours for granted. They are worth a lifetime.

Mark 5:22-24 (NIV)

Then one of the synagogue leaders, named Jairus, came, and when he saw Jesus, he fell at his feet. He pleaded earnestly with him, "My little daughter is dying. Please come and put your hands on her so that she will be healed and live." So Jesus went with him. While Jesus was still speaking, some people came from the house of Jairus, the synagogue leader. "Your daughter is dead," they said. "Why bother the teacher anymore?" Overhearing what they said, Jesus told him, "Don't be afraid; just believe."

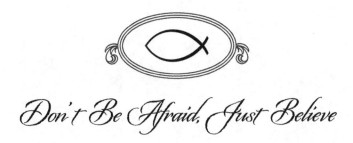

Don't Be Afraid, Just Believe

Jairus was a man of influence in his community. His money and power could give him just about anything he wanted. Yet he was desperate. Jairus had other attributes. He had enough wisdom to know that his money and influence could not heal the person he loved.

He reached out to the only one who had the power to restore life to his daughter. Jesus. Jesus healed this young girl without even directly touching the girl. Jesus later told the people "Don't be afraid; just believe."

Jesus is saying the same words to you. Don't be afraid; Just believe. Miracles still happen and God is still willing to perform them for you. Just Believe.

Deuteronomy 4:9 (NLT)

"But watch out! Be careful never to forget what you yourself have seen. Do not let these memories escape from your mind as long as you live! And be sure to pass them on to your children and grandchildren.

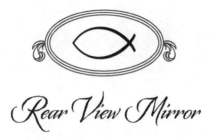

Rear View Mirror

As TIME GOES BY FOR YOU there may be a lot of opportunities to be alone with your thoughts. You will remember how it all started. You will be able to look in the rear view mirror and dredge up the time and place when you were told you had cancer. You will remember some things and for other things you will have no recollection.

The rear view mirror allows us to see what is behind us. We can see who and what is following us. We can see the exit ramp that we missed. A great purpose for the rear view mirror is that it enables us to see that God has moved us forward using the rear view mirror as proof that something is behind us. Praise God!

Many say to forget the past. I say remember the past to add to the testimony that God is building for you right now. Whatever the outcome, whatever the treatment plan you have a testimony right now. Each day you are fighting, hoping, trusting and believing, you are building and living your testimony.

So, remember the past, build your testimony on your past. Know that you have a rear view mirror. Don't live in the past but don't forget what God has brought you through, for it will give strength to another person.

1 Thessalonians 5:18 (NLT)

*Be thankful in all circumstances, for this is God's
will for you who belong to Christ Jesus.*

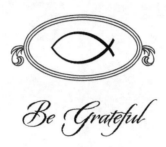

Be Grateful

I SAY BE GRATEFUL. "YOUR RESPONSE may be what do I have to be grateful for? I would not wish this on my worst enemy." Let me share this fact with you. Being grateful has nothing to do with the specific situation but has everything to do with Christ and your relationship with Him.

Be grateful because you may be experiencing one of the greatest opportunities in your life to see God work in ways where people will marvel at His power. Be grateful because you will learn to rely and trust in God like you've never had before. This time is an opportunity for you to reflex and trust that what God has planned for you is greater than the current circumstances. You will feel his presence if you allow the Holy Spirit to come in and engulf you.

Gratefulness helps you to remember that you have a deep dependence on Him and nothing can be done outside of Him and nothing should be attempted without Him.

Genesis 28:15 (NLT)

"What's more, I am with you, and I will protect you wherever you go. One day I will bring you back to this land. I will not leave you until I have finished giving you everything I have promised you."

Do It Now

YOU WERE CREATED FOR A PURPOSE. One day you were born and one day you will die. In between that time you will live your life. You will make decisions, both good and bad, you will show love and received love, you will have regrets about the past and hopes for the future.

One day you will wake up and you will take seriously that life is fleeting. That one day you will run out of time to do everything you wanted to do, say everything you wanted to say. There really are not enough hours in the day....and yet you are still here.

You are still here therefore you have the time now, RIGHT NOW, to say what you've always wanted to say. To say I'm sorry, I love you, Thank you. DO IT NOW! You will never have this day again and may not have the opportunity to hug her, kiss him, forgive them.

You are here today...but THEIR tomorrow is not promised.

Romans 12:12 (NLT)

Rejoice in our confident hope. Be patient in trouble, and keep on praying.

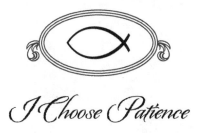

I Choose Patience

Today I will take one day at a time. I will not try to rush what will happen tomorrow nor will I worry about what tomorrow will bring. The word of God says tomorrow has trouble of its own. I am here today. Therefore I will deal with the things of today. The things I deal with today are enough. I trust God will take of tomorrow.

Today I will have patience when I feel a sense of eagerness. I will choose patience when I feel myself trying to "step in" for God. I will ask for patience when I need to know NOW!

Today I will practice patience as if my life depended on it. I know waiting on God can be difficult but today I will wait and tomorrow I will wait and trust. The next day I will start all over with patience and trust.

I choose patience.

Joshua 24:15 NIV

But if serving the LORD seems undesirable to you, then choose for yourselves this day whom you will serve, whether the gods your ancestors served beyond the Euphrates, or the gods of the Amorites, in whose land you are living. But as for me and my household, we will serve the LORD."

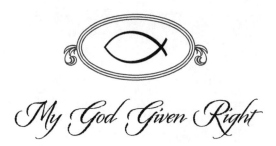

My God Given Right

I CHOOSE THE MOST HIGH GOD. It's a good thing that God designed us and gave us choices. I have the God given right to choose to believe in God or reject God. We must all remember that the choice to serve and worship God is so necessary and reasonable that any other choice pales to this. Worshiping anything else would be in vain.

Chapter 24 in the book of Joshua he was trying to explain to the people that they do have a choice. The wise choice and the best choice is God. As faithful Christians God is our ONLY choice. For we know of the love God has for us even when we are at our worst. Make your choice carefully. Your creator desires a relationship with you. But He also desires that you choose Him and trust him in every aspect of your life.

Choosing to trust in a doctor, medicine, treatments or even your family is not the answer. God only provided all of these things to help you and to assist you, He blesses you with these people and things to show His love for you. He can even perform miracles through these vehicles.

Use Wisdom...Choose God.

Jeremiah 17:7 (NLT)

"But blessed are those who trust in the Lord and have made the Lord their hope and confidence.

God Is Getting Ready To Bless You

THE KEY TO REALLY UNDERSTANDING THE blessings of God is that the blessing is already waiting for you. It is already prepared for you and God is just waiting for the right timing to blow your mind!

Your blessing is already in place for you. God would like to lay out the red carpet for you. He wants to keep you encouraged and in a mindset of hopefulness. These blessing will be given to you because of you, in spite of you and simply out of love. No one can dismiss these blessing but you. No one can reject these blessing but you. In the midst of your situation God is still blessing you. Blessings come in all forms.

Being consumed with your recovery, treatment and surgery can make you doubt that you are still being blessed. However, your blessings may come in the form of a financial windfall to pay for medication, finding a nurse who loves her job and takes a special interest in you or even a treatment schedule that is perfect for you to regain normalcy to life. God is blessing you right now!

John 6:68 (NLT)

Simon Peter replied, "Lord, to whom would we go?
You have the words that give eternal life.

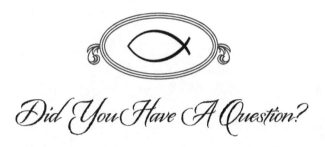

Did You Have A Question?

THERE ARE SEVERAL PEOPLE WHO COMPLAINED or called out to God about an illness or a physical condition. Moses, David, Job and even Jeremiah soon found out that God was not only there in the good days but also in the dark days.

God is not upset when you ask questions about your pain and diagnosis. He does not punish his children for wanting to know the reasons for things that happen. Curiosity and questioning is part of our makeup. He listens, cares and lifts them out of their diversity in His perfect time.

He gives mercy to those who are suffering and victory to those who feel hopeless. Nothing you go through will be wasted. For God will use it all to help you be stronger in faith and to help others.

2 Thessalonians 1:3 (NLT)

*Dear brothers and sisters, we can't help but thank God for you, because
your faith is flourishing and your love for one another is growing.*

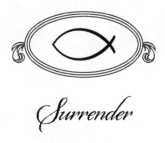

Surrender

TRY THIS. TRY PRAYING FOR SOMEONE else with cancer. I know your focus is on you right now. You feel bad. This may be one of the worst times in your life if not the worst time. But have you tried praying for others who are going through the same thing you are going through. You, better than anyone, know what they may be feeling and what they are dealing with.

One of the best things we can do for another person with cancer is to pray for them. Whether you believe it or not people are praying for you. People you will never meet are praying fervently and continually for you. These people know that prayer is critical to your healing and to your attitude toward your condition.

Something ALWAYS happens when we pray. God will either show mercy, give us grace bless someone else, etc. etc. No prayer is ever in vain. Our prayers is our way of saying to God that we know we don't have the power to deal with, solve or change a situation and that we need Him to intervene according to His will. Our heavenly Father is not one who leaves us when we need him the most. He hears and He cares and He's working it out for our good. Surrender it all to Him in prayer.

You do what you know how to do and God will do the rest.

John 13:17 (NLT)

Now that you know these things, God will bless you for doing them.

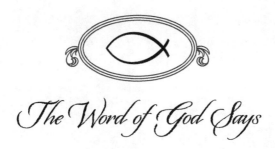

The Word of God Says

1. Peace I leave with you; my peace I give you. I do not give to you as the world gives. Do not let your heats be troubled and do not be afraid. John 14:27

2. Though you have made me see troubles, many and bitter, you will restore my life again from the depths of the earth you will again bring me up. Psalms 71:20

3. If anyone of you lacks wisdom, he should ask God, who gives generously to all without finding fault, and it will be given to him. But when he asks, he must believe and not doubt, because he who doubts is like a wave of the sea, blown and tossed by the wind. James 1:5-6

4. Though I walk in the midst of trouble, you preserve my life you stretch out your hand against the anger of my foes, with your right hand you save me. Psalms 138:7

Philippians 4:12-13 (NIV)

I know what it is to be in need, and I know what it is to have plenty. I have learned the secret of being content in any and every situation, whether well fed or hungry, whether living in plenty or in want. I can do all this through him who gives me strength.

A Prayer Away

THIS JOURNEY YOU ARE ON COULD cause some to fall into a state of depression. You have to be very careful. It is not God's will for you to be depressed nor hopeless.

If you start to have a spirit of depression it is time to speak hope to your situation by being grateful for what you do have. Write down the things you are grateful for. Nothing is too small to write down and nothing is too obvious. You have much to be grateful for in your life. Start with your senses. Be grateful for the gift of hearing, for touch, for sight. Continue with your material possessions, your family, friends and pets. Continue the list with the blessings God gave you in the past and continue with the blessings you are asking for in the future.

Depression is not of God and is a spirit that must be defeated by the power of God. Help is available and waiting but you must open your mouth and share your sorrow with someone you trust. The first one to help you will always be God and he will lead you in the right direction to receive help whether it is a therapist or doctor. Hope is always a prayer away.

1 Samuel 3:10 (NIV)

*The Lord came and stood there, calling as at
the other times, "Samuel! Samuel!"
Then Samuel said, "Speak, for your servant is listening."*

Speak Lord

Is GOD SPEAKING TO YOU BY allowing this journey in your life? What is He trying to say to you? While Samuel was lying down God called him three times. Before Eli told him that the Lord was calling him. God was trying to get his attention because He was trying to tell him something. When God is trying to get your attention it will sometimes be in ways that are unconventional or even ways that you will not expect.

God wants your attention because there is clearly something God has for you or wants you to know. It will affect you or someone else but God has decided to deliver the message, the miracle, His will through you. He must first get your attention.

When you hear Him, simply say...Speak Lord your servant is listening.

1 Peter 1:21 (NLT)

Through Christ you have come to trust in God. And you have placed your faith and hope in God because he raised Christ from the dead and gave him great glory.

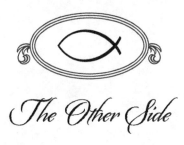

The Other Side

IF OR WHEN YOU EXPERIENCE CHEMOTHERAPY or radiation you will discover that you will not be able to control everything you once were able to control. You will just not be physically able to do everything. Your mind will be in so many different directions that there are not enough hours in the day to deal with the same agenda you did before this journey. Things change after a diagnosis of cancer. All things do not have to be negative.

When Saul became Paul he went through a total mind and heart transformation. This experience he had on the road to Damascus transformed how he thought and how he saw his future. He knew he could not go back to the same old agenda and the same control over his life that he once had. He realized that his time and his will was now in the hands of God. He accepted that and trusted God would help him endure through the process of change and come out on the winning side.

Habakkuk 2:3 (NLT)

This vision is for a future time. It describes the end, and it will be fulfilled. If it seems slow in coming, wait patiently, for it will surely take place. It will not be delayed

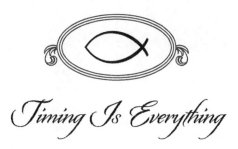

Timing Is Everything

MY MOTHER BATTLED THREE DIFFERENT TYPES of cancer. She is the strongest women I have ever known. She was courageous and had always said what she felt. Sometimes her truth would make us laugh. She could be funny even when she was not trying to be funny. She was the type of person who made her own decisions and no one was able to control her. She knew God existed and talked to Him daily. My fondest memory of my mother is when we prayed together. She fought and endured until God called her home.

It was not easy for her but she did what she had to do until she didn't have to do it any longer. She is now resting and waiting for her Savior to return and take her to her final destination which is heaven. It's not over yet. The pain on this earth has passed for her but she will now be escorted to her eternal home that has been prepared for her.

We will all be in a position when God will call us home. It will not be premature nor will it be exactly how we plan it because it is not our role to decide when and where but it is Gods' decision on the date when our bodies will no longer be productive. Trust God in His divine timing.

Titus 3:4-6 (NLT)

When God our Savior revealed his kindness and love, he saved us, not because of the righteous things we had done, but because of his mercy. He washed away our sins, giving us a new birth and new life through the Holy Spirit. He generously poured out the Spirit upon us through Jesus Christ our Savior.

Shared Experiences

OVER TWO THOUSAND YEARS AGO GOD decided to come to us as a man who had the power and the purpose to save us from ourselves. He came to us in a vulnerable body that could be bruised. He prayed to the Father for what he needed and wanted during his journey. Jesus felt pain, rejection and betrayal. What Jesus went through was not in vain and something great came out of his agony. He went through it willingly because he trusted that the Father knew the plans for his life.

Nothing you go through will be in vain. God does not always bring things to us but he does allow things in our life. If you are a child of God you are under the protection of God. You are under the divine will of the Creator and He will not leave you out there on your own to fight this fight. Jesus may not have had cancer but he knows exactly how you feel and what you're going through. Talk to him about it. He has experience in wanting what is best for you.

1 Chronicles 4:10 (NLT)

He was the one who prayed to the God of Israel, "Oh, that you would bless me and expand my territory! Please be with me in all that I do, and keep me from all trouble and pain!" And God granted him his request.

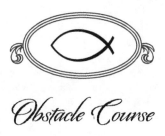

Obstacle Course

THIS JOURNEY YOU ARE ON IS an obstacle course. An obstacle course is simply a variety of physical obstacles that one navigates. Sometimes an obstacle course includes a mental test. We think of an obstacle course as a race or possibly a part of a competition. While tackling the obstacle course you will jump, walk, balance, breathe fast, breathe slow, focus, run and even get tired. Throughout the course, some of the obstacles may seem too enormous to tackle or you may seem to run out of energy.

How do you get to the finish line? You just keep going. You take one step at a time, you ask God for more energy to finish the race. You pace yourself and you look at the obstacles as a mountain that only God can move. Cancer thinks it has you. The truth is that your God has it. God is all-powerful and has power over any obstacle you are up against.

Zechariah 13:8-9 (NLT)

Two-thirds of the people in the land will be cut off and die,"
says the Lord. "But one-third will be left in the land.
I will bring that group through the fire and make them pure.
I will refine them like silver and purify them like gold. They
will call on my name, and I will answer them. I will say, 'These
are my people,' and they will say, 'The Lord is our God.'

Get Prepared Through Prayer

IF GOD ALLOWS TRIALS AND TROUBLES in your life you can get prepared for it through prayer. You can ask God to help you to deal with the trials with wisdom and courage. To have the strength to endure and to show you a way out. Prayer will acknowledge that God is in control and show your reliance on His strength in every situation.

Nowhere in the bible does it say that we will not have troubles. In fact, the bible says in John 16:33, In this world you will have troubles. Prayer is a way of reaching God before the trouble reaches you. When you pray you are preparing your heart and your spirit to receive whatever He has for you. Receive His grace, His peace, His wisdom. Your heart is expecting it because you prayed for it.

1 John 5:14-15 (NLT)

And we are confident that he hears us whenever we ask for anything that pleases him. And since we know he hears us when we make our requests, we also know that he will give us what we ask for.

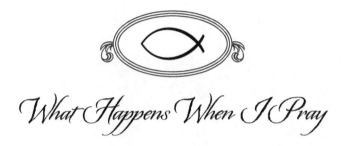

What Happens When I Pray

IF YOU'VE NEVER HAD A CONSISTENT and healthy prayer life you are about to now. There may be times that you are so mentally and physically weak that all you can handle is to pray. The fact of the matter is that prayer is the most important thing you can do. As you continue to pray and seek God in prayer your faith will grow. That faith is exactly what you need now. As your faith grows God will show you that he does not change but you will.

You will change how you see the situation. You will change your attitude about what you are going through. God ordains prayer as the vehicle by which he accomplishes His will. God acts through prayer not apart from it. Therefore, God will do many things if you pray. You have nothing to lose in prayer.

Galatians 2:20 (NLT)

*My old self has been crucified with Christ. It is no longer I who live,
but Christ lives in me. So, I live in this earthly body by trusting
in the Son of God, who loved me and gave himself for me.*

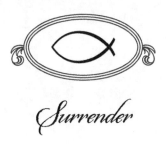

Surrender

Try this. Try praying for someone else with cancer. I know your focus is on your right now. You feel bad and need everything you can to get to the next day. This may be one of the worst times in your life if not the worst time. But have you tried praying for others who are going through the same thing you are going through? You know, better than most, what they may be feeling and what they are dealing with.

God's word tells us to pray for one another. While we are praying for others, we are not focused on ourselves. We are not focused on what can go wrong with us or how bad things may look for ourselves. We are focused on carrying each other's burdens. Galatians 6:2 states "Carry each other's burdens, and in this way you will fulfill the law of Christ."

The prayer of a righteous man carries much weight. Someone else needs your prayers. Remember there is someone else praying for you.

James 1:5 (NLT)

*If you need wisdom, ask our generous God, and he will
give it to you. He will not rebuke you for asking.*

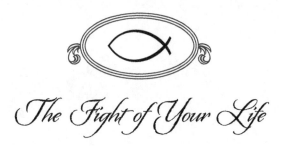

The Fight of Your Life

YOU ARE IN THE FIGHT FOR your life. It is said that you truly know who your friends are when you are at the worst times in your life. You will find many people who are going to be very supportive to you, even strangers. Then you may also receive comments from many who think they are being helpful by telling you the stories about the many people who have died from cancer and how horrible it is. You will get unsolicited medical advice. Some may even ask or insinuate that you brought this on yourself due to sin or other habits. Some of these people mean well. Others do not.

I have found the best advice came from those who had already been in the fight. Individuals who traveled the same road but had different journeys and shared their experiences with me. These people were invaluable. Their comments are priceless when you're in the fight of your life. Allow the Holy Spirit to lead you to who you should talk to and who you should listen to.

Nehemiah 9:6 (NLT)

"You alone are the Lord. You made the skies and the heavens and all the stars. You made the earth and the seas and everything in them. You preserve them all, and the angels of heaven worship you.

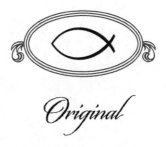

Original

IT IS TRUE, AS SOMEONE ONCE said, "We need to live as if everything depends on God and work as if everything depends on us." Why is it that we forget that we are the product of and the creation of God? The creator knows when the creation is not functioning as intended and needs adjustments.

Would you go to a doctor to fix your car? Would you seek out a grocer to build your house? Of course not. You would go to the specialist, the creator to seek guidance and restoration. Because you are an original you need to go to the one who has the original blueprints.

You were created in love and that alone is what God continues to have for you. Go to the one who loves you.

Revelation 14:13 (NLT)

*And I heard a voice from heaven saying, "Write this down:
Blessed are those who die in the Lord from now on. Yes, says
the Spirit, they are blessed indeed, for they will rest from
their hard work; for their good deeds follow them!"*

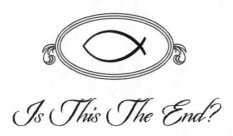

Is This The End?

ONLY GOD KNOWS THE FUTURE. ONLY God knows when you will die. As a child of the King it is important to know that God has a plan for you and His holy will is all about what is best for you because He loves you enough to protect you and bless you.

Passing away from the effects of Cancer is only one way to say that the body needs rest; that the Father has decided to call you home. Cancer does not win. Victory is going home to be with the Lord, in God's perfect timing.

God may heal you or God may not heal you. Either way, it is important to remember that God be glorified in both situations. God is glorified in healing and God can be glorified by the testimony of your salvation with the assurance of being with God in eternity.

Death is nothing to fear. It is only a part of life.

Hebrews 4:12 (NLT)

For the word of God is alive and powerful. It is sharper than the sharpest two-edged sword, cutting soul and spirit, between joint and marrow. It exposes our innermost thoughts and desires.

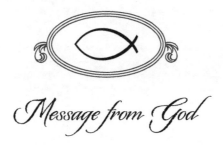

Message from God

Dear Child,

I AM WATCHING EVERYTHING THAT IS happening to you. I see the pain. I hear the questions. I also have a plan that is designed uniquely for you. This trial you are going through right now is just that; a trial. This journey is one that others have traveled but your road is paved with obstacles that only you can travel. It must be this way because the blessings you will receive from this journey are created only for you.

My wisdom is mysterious to you, I know. Trust it. It will lead you in the right direction and help you to be victorious in ways that you cannot imagine right now. Keep your focus on me. I am the Way, the Truth and the Light. This light will lead you in to my will. The Truth will enable you to get through each day. The Way will guide you to the solutions you are seeking.

Take delight in the miracles I will give you each day. Even on the days that are difficult for you, I am working on your behalf to bring peace to your spirit.

Take courage. I am with you even to the end of the earth.

Love,
Father, Son, Holy Spirit

John 10:10 (NLT)

*The thief's purpose is to steal and kill and destroy. My
purpose is to give them a rich and satisfying life.*

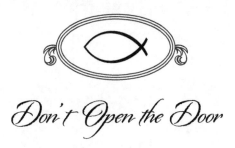

Don't Open the Door

SATAN WILL START TO KNOCK AT your door. He will remind you of everything that you did wrong in the past. He will remind you of your lies, your bad deeds. He will throw the sin of your past in your face to discourage you and to make you think that God has abandoned you. He will want you to think that you are going through this because you are not loved. He will use everything at his disposal to try and turn you away from your God.

DON'T FALL FOR IT!

God has not forsaken you and He does not hate you. God loves you and just as Jesus had to go through something on earth. So do you. No, you are not Jesus but you belong to Him. You are one of his servants and just like he was maligned, hated and persecuted so the same Satan is doing to you. God has not left you out there on your own. Don't believe the lies.

Don't fall for it!

Ezra 10:12 (NLT)

*Then the whole assembly raised their voices and answered,
"Yes, you are right; we must do as you say!"*

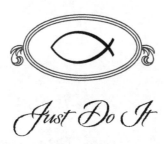

Just Do It

GOD HAS A LOT TO SAY to us in His word. He tells us what to do and when to do it. God is not a mystical figure that only cares about himself. You were created in love because God wanted to love you. Doing what God wants us to do is showing love in return. His commands are ways to protect us just because of that love. Think about it. He tells us to love one another. With everything that we must deal with in this world would it not be easier if we just loved one another? He tells us to forgive one another. If we did, we would let go of a lot of stress and anger.

Life is hard enough and life is short. Why hold on to anger and hatred through unforgiveness? Unforgiveness and holding on to that anger only hurts you not the other person. It is time to take care of you by forgiving them. Let it go. Be healed and start living.

Malachi 3:16-18 (MSG)

Then those whose lives honored GOD got together and talked it over. GOD saw what they were doing and listened in. A book was opened in God's presence and minutes were taken of the meeting, with the names of the GOD-fearers written down, all the names of those who honored GOD's name. GOD-of-the-Angel-Armies said, "They're mine, all mine. They'll get special treatment when I go into action. I treat them with the same consideration and kindness that parents give the child who honors them. Once more you'll see the difference it makes between being a person who does the right thing and one who doesn't, between serving God and not serving him."

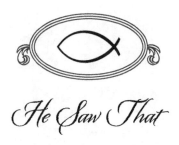

He Saw That

No matter where you find yourself in life continue to honor God. Continue to lift Him up in good times and in bad. God does see and acknowledges you when you serve him. God can see how you are treated by others and the ones who care about you. It is not your job to worry or stress over others and what is going on outside of your control. What is in your control is the power to worship and continue to live a life of faith. Show the world that even in your weakest hour you still believe and still know who is in control.

Song of Solomon 2:11 (NLT)

Look, the winter is past, and the rains are over and gone.

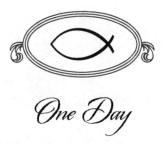

One Day

ONE DAY IT WILL BE ALL over. God wants it that way. Everything in this life is temporary. The troubles of this world will be over. The questions, the doubt will all be in the past. In Gods' own timing and divine plan, things will go exactly as He allows it.

The sufferings of this day will all come to an end and perfection will be waiting for us. The suffering you have and know now will one day be in the past. The winter is past and the rains are over and gone.

Leviticus 8:10-12 (NLT)

Then Moses took the anointing oil and anointed the Tabernacle and everything in it, making them holy. He sprinkled the oil on the altar seven times, anointing it and all its utensils, as well as the washbasin and its stand, making them holy. Then he poured some of the anointing oil on Aaron's head, anointing him and making him holy for his work.

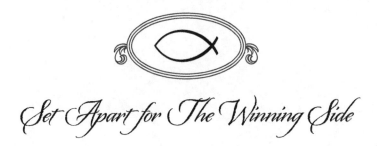

Set Apart for The Winning Side

To be consecrated means to set apart to the service of a deity. As a servant of The Most High God you have been set apart from the world to fulfill the will of God. You have a purpose and while living out that purpose you will come against some ungodly things. Some things will be to divert your attention away from your purpose and His plan. Don't worry, God has planted in you the Holy Spirit that will enable you to overcome anything that may come your way. The scripture encourages us to not fear anything.

God is stronger than whatever Satan may throw your way. Remember that Satan is already defeated and he knows it. He must do everything he can to deter you, to slow you down. Just remember that you have been set apart and chosen by God for His service. There is no better side to be on than the winning side.

Jude 1:2 (NLT)

May God give you more and more mercy, peace, and love.

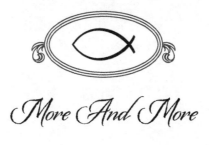

More And More

THERE WILL BE TIMES IN YOUR life when you will need something more than the regular day to day help or inspiration or even advice. This point in your life may be one of them. You need more help than normal, more advice than you normally ask for. You may seek out people that you have not talked to in a while who you know have what you may need. Needing help and asking for help is not weak. It is being strong. If God wanted us to live on this earth alone without anyone He could have made an earth for each individual person to exist on his own.

God actually wants to give you more and more of Him. As much of Him as you can handle at any point in your life. He wants so badly to fill you with His spirit because that is where the love is. That is the part where he can and will connect with you.

He wants to show his mercy because that's the kind of God He is. He is continually showing you grace only because of His love for you. There is no one else on this earth or beyond that can and does love you like God!

Luke 10:34 (NLT)

Going over to him, the Samaritan soothed his wounds with olive oil and wine and bandaged them. Then he put the man on his own donkey and took him to an inn, where he took care of him.

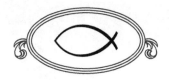

Modern Medicine and Miracles

GOD'S HEALING POWER IS MIRACULOUS. GOD can heal and deliver anyway He wants. Sometimes God uses the blessing of medicine to heal what ails us. Medicine is just one way God has chosen to deliver healing to us. Luke who was a writer of one of the gospels in the bible was a physician. He even advised one of his students, Timothy, about the use of medicine to help the sick.

God gave us medicine to help us, however, we must also be careful to not misuse these substances. Our bodies are the temple of God in which we must use them to the glory of God. That includes what we put on it and in it.

God provides for us through many modern-day advancements. Technology, medical science and treatments get better every day. This, however, should never be a substitute for our trust and guidance of the Holy Spirit. Let the Spirit lead you in wisdom and knowledge when making decisions about modern-day medicine.

Mark 1:17 (NLT)

Jesus called out to them, "Come, follow me, and I will show you how to fish for people!"

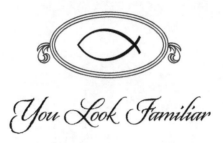

You Look Familiar

THE CROSS IS LIKELY THE MOST well-known. You are also a symbol of the Christian faith. The Cross is likely the most well-known. You are also a symbol of Christian faith. Your attitude, your prayer life, your comments, reactions, speech and even your priorities in life speak to who you are and what you believe in.

Some will be able to look at you and know that you have a deeper sense of who you are beyond who others think you are. That is the essence of your symbol. That symbol is your life, how you live it and how you respond to situations that happen to you.

Everyone who wears a cross around their neck is not always a Christian, everyone who attends church is not saved and washed cleaned by the blood of Christ. Let your life and light shine as a symbol of who your God is in spite of your circumstances. Your witness, your life, your symbol is as much a testimony as anything else.

Ephesians 6:13-18 (MSG)

Be prepared. You're up against far more than you can handle on your own. Take all the help you can get, every weapon God has issued, so that when it's all over but the shouting you'll still be on your feet. Truth, righteousness, peace, faith, and salvation are more than words. Learn how to apply them. You'll need them throughout your life. God's Word is an indispensable weapon. In the same way, prayer is essential in this ongoing warfare. Pray hard and long. Pray for your brothers and sisters. Keep your eyes open. Keep each other's spirits up so that no one falls behind or drops out.

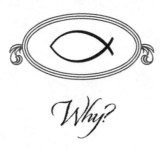

Why?

You ask the question "Why does God allow sickness at all?" This is a difficult question and the complete answer can only come from God. However, there are things we do know. We know that God always wants what's best for us. We also know that we live in physical bodies that have diseases, are full of sin and eventually die.

Yes, it is true God does allow things. It is to accomplish His sovereign purpose. It is during the times of sickness that we really rely on God. We are forced to rest our minds and bodies to think, meditate and reflex. We'll ask a lot of questions and are still enough to wait and listen for the answers. Sickness forces us to look at the frailties of life.

Only God knows truly why He does what He does. It is our assignment to continue to be disciples with the questions and unknown futures. We know who holds all the answers. Let's trust in Him.

Ezekiel 37:14 (NLT)

I will put my Spirit in you, and you will live again and return home to your own land. Then you will know that I, the Lord, have spoken, and I have done what I said. Yes, the Lord has spoken!

Reality

Here's the reality of things.

They made Him carry the heavy cross

They hung God's son on a tree

They drove nails through his hands and feet.

They pierced Him in his side

The people cried and some cheered.

He still said "Father forgive them".

People left Him there to die.

But it was not the end. For in three days he would rise and our debt for everything we did or would do was paid. All because he died.

There's a spirit in you that enables you to live a new life.

He died so you could live an abundant life. Don't you dare give up on God. The price for you was high!

Judges 6:23 (NIV)

But the Lord said to him, "Peace! Do not be afraid. You are not going to die.

What Does God Know About Me?

To be in the presence of God is a humbling experience. Lying in a hospital bed is also a humbling experience. One thing is for sure, when you are lying in a hospital bed you want the presence of God in that room. In that room a lot of things happen. Words are said that are shocking. The words, "you are dying, you are going to die, death is imminent" is a daunting moment. No matter how you phrase the words they still give you a knot in your throat. A pit in your stomach.

What if you hear the words "You are not going to die?" Does it present another set of feelings?

No one can tell you when you are going to die. Only God knows. Doctors can tell you what they think may happen. They, however, do not know the date or time. Only God knows. Keep the details in Gods' hands. Don't allow man to be the timer for your life.

2 Chronicles 9:6 (NLT)

I didn't believe what was said until I arrived here and saw it with my own eyes. In fact, I had not heard the half of your great wisdom! It is far beyond what I was told.

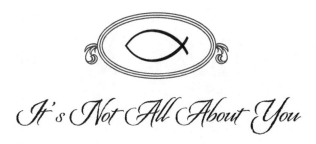

It's Not All About You

I LOVE THE PHRASE "YOU DON'T look like what you've been through". Individuals may say this about you or even to you. If they only knew the full story. When one hears that a loved one has cancer there are dozens of emotions they will feel. Your cancer journey affects more than you.

Your miracle of healing, the suffering, what happened, how it happened and even why it happened may all be the topic of conversation among people you know and those you do not know.

Your report will amaze people. It will give people hope. Your report will encourage those who feel they are losing the fight. No matter what state you are in be prepared to give a report of faith and hope.

2 John 1:12 (NLT)

I have much more to say to you, but I don't want to do it with paper and ink. For I hope to visit you soon and talk with you face to face. Then our joy will be complete.

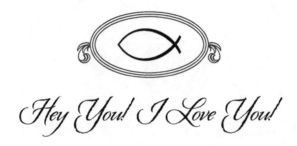

Hey You! I Love You!

IN THIS DAY OF THE INTERNET and modern technology we can reach others in a matter of seconds at any time of the day. Nothing takes the place of someone being with you face to face. Their touch, seeing their smile or even connecting by looking in a persons' eye makes a difference.

Whenever you get the opportunity to say I love you face to face, do so. You will never know when you will see them again or even if it will be the last time. Jesus spent time alone with God and with his disciples. Jesus understood the importance of relationships and took the time to show love and to say how much He loved. There is no substitute for the words I Love You!

Joel 2:21 (NLT)

Don't be afraid, O land. Be glad now and rejoice,
for the Lord has done great things.

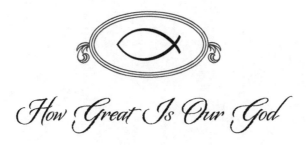

How Great Is Our God

MEDITATE ON THE GREAT THINGS GOD has done for you. Surely there are things you are thankful for. Even now. Rejoice in those things. Satan will always try and make you believe that your situation is who you are. Remember, Satan is a liar. That's who he is and that's what he does. He wants you to forget the good God has done for you. More important he wants you to believe that God will no longer bless you or be with you. Rebuke Satan in the name of Jesus.

God loves you and is the same God yesterday, today and tomorrow. Rejoice in the fact that he does not change and he will continue to do great things for you and through you according to His will.

Colossians 3:13 (NLT)

*Make allowance for each other's faults, and forgive anyone who offends
you. Remember, the Lord forgave you, so you must forgive others.*

Forgiven

FORGIVENESS IS NOT ONLY A COMMANDMENT it is a source of freedom. You have more to concentrate on now and unforgiveness should not be on the agenda.

One thing about forgiveness is that it allows you to move forward in your life. Don't worry about an apology from someone for you to forgive them. You may never get one. Your forgiveness should not depend on their apology. Your obedience is what matters. W Why is obedience the topic? Obedience is always the key to the blessings of God to flow in your life. Forgive them for you. You don't need negative energy in your life right now. Forgive and move on. Forgiveness does not mean that you condone what has been done to you. Forgiveness means that you have let go of the hurt and move forward in love toward the offender.

When you forgive that is one less burden you have to deal with. This journey is full of a lot of baggage. You do not need one more bag to carry. Let it go and get on with your life.

Esther 4:14 (NLT)

If you keep quiet at a time like this, deliverance and relief for the Jews will arise from some other place, but you and your relatives will die. Who knows if perhaps you were made queen for just such a time as this?"

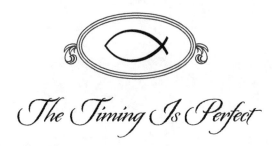

The Timing Is Perfect

QUEEN ESTHER HAD SOME DECISIONS TO make. Would she speak up and do something to save her people or would she remain silent? Both options bring consequences. The scripture eludes to the fact that God allowed her to be in a certain position for the exact time in order to work out God's plan for His people.

There will be a time when you will have an opportunity to do the work of God, to testify about God, to encourage someone through their journey.

Have you thought about your purpose? Have you considered how you can use this portion of your life story to encourage others, lift God up or even grow from this?

Be bold, open your mouth. Who knows, you may have come to this position for such a time as this.

Acts 1:7 (NLT)

He replied, "The Father alone has the authority to set those dates and times, and they are not for you to know."

What Time Is It?

YOU WILL NOT RECEIVE AN ANSWER to every question that you will have. Some questions will be answered for you by human knowledge. Some will be answered by Godly wisdom. Some questions will not be answered. In God's infinite wisdom, He knows there are some things you do not need to know. There are things that only God is privy to. Living under the authority of God and His wisdom is a great place to be.

Nehemiah 1:4 (NLT)

*When I heard this, I sat down and wept. In fact, for days I
mourned, fasted, and prayed to the God of heaven.*

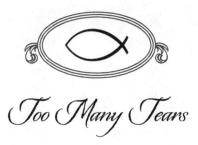

Too Many Tears

FOR MANY, TEARS ARE PLENTIFUL DURING this time, even in recovery. Some tears are even full of joy. When you sit back and collect the thoughts that once ran through your head and now you discover you are on the other end of those thoughts. A place you did not know if you would get to. A place where you thought was so far away you dare not dream of a better day. You were just trying to take it day by day.

Cancer is not always an immediate death. Yet when we announce we have cancer some think that it is the end of our time here on earth. There are so many advancements in medicine and options for treatments than there has ever been in the past.

There is something that stands above treatments and medical advancements that God enables us to have access to. It is called miracles. Yes, miracles still are in style. God still perform miracles every day. I have never discounted the ability of God to perform miracles in my life. A miracle could come in any form at any time.

Philemon 1:22 (NLT)

One more thing—please prepare a guest room for me, for I am hoping that God will answer your prayers and let me return to you soon.

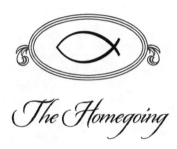

The Homegoing

GET READY! YOU ARE RETURNING TO your family, your friends and much more after one of the most serious times of your life. You have just been told something or went through something that is life-changing.

Let me warn you that your life may be a bit different. The way you look at situations and people may be different. Life will seem more precious, time more priceless. Family members will be easier to forgive and enemies will not get as much attention. Things you once took for granted will be important. You will deal with others differently because you were reminded how precious life is.

A room is being prepared for you. God has answered your prayers.

Lamentations 3:22 (NLT)

The faithful love of the Lord never ends! His mercies never cease.

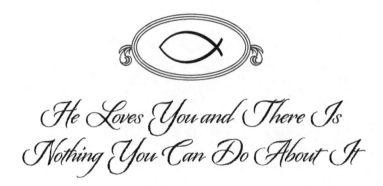

He Loves You and There Is Nothing You Can Do About It

GOD'S LOVE NEVER ENDS. THERE IS nothing you can do and nothing you can say to make God's love for you change. This is one of the joys of life. To know that God loves you even with all your mistakes and flaws. He loves you while you were yet a sinner.

Imagine what your life would be like without God. Yes, it would be hell! God loves you enough to die for you so that you would not have to experience hell. That love is greater than anything that tries to destroy you. Including cancer. Cancer is nothing in the hands of God.

Hosea 6:2 (NIV)

*After two days he will revive us; on the third day he
will restore us, that we may live in his presence.*

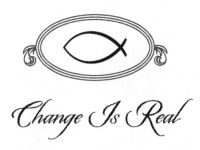

Change Is Real

TIMING IS EVERYTHING. REST IS EXTREMELY important. You don't have to have cancer to adopt this piece of wisdom. Doing things when your mind is ready but your body is not has proven to be an unwise combination.

The bible says there is a season for everything. This is your season to take care of you. Time to spend more time with God, talking with God, reading the word of God. This is a season to reevaluate your relationship with God and others. A season to decide on changes for your life.

Be deliberate about the changes knowing they will bring you closer to your God. Don't apologize for the changes as they will make you better to serve your God.

Life is short. Take advantage of every minute and live life on purpose!

3 John 1:4 (NLT)

*I could have no greater joy than to hear that
my children are following the truth.*

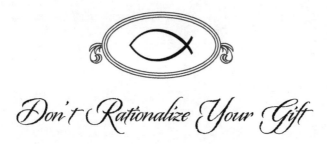

Don't Rationalize Your Gift

WHAT IS YOUR TRUTH? AS CHRISTIANS our truth is found in Jesus Christ. God is beyond happy to know that we walk each day knowing and believing in who He is and that we know He loves us by dying for us. As Christians that is our truth. He is the Way, the Truth and the Life.

If we keep this truth in our mind, heart and spirit it will sustain us even in the worst of times.

How? Consider this: Jesus Christ did not die for us to live a life of hopelessness or a life of constant fear, agony and struggle. Yes, there will be hard times and for some, horrible times. However, God gives us something during these times that will help us get through. That "something" is peace.

That peace He gives us passes all understanding. Don't try to rationalize it. It doesn't come from human knowledge. Don't try to extend it. It is given by Grace.

Receive it just as it is given. With love, from above.

Isaiah 40:31 (NLT)

But those who trust in the Lord will find new strength. They will soar high on wings like eagles. They will run and not grow weary. They will walk and not faint.

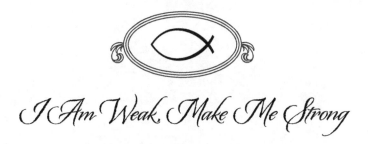

I Am Weak, Make Me Strong

WHEN WE THINK OF WEAKNESSES, WE see it as physical, mental and even a spiritual manifestation. Dealing with any form of cancer can affect you in all of these ways. Your strength takes a brutal hit and what you were once able to do now becomes a struggle. This is the time when God is calling on us to call on Him. God knew that we would have moments of weakness and this has come as no surprise to Him. God has already prepared the answer. He accounted for your need of hope and strength.

God wants us to put our hope in Him for our daily strength. The strength we receive will come in many forms. Do not discount the package your deliverance comes in!

Remember that His timing is perfect and He is our strength in times of weakness. Our hope and strength are found in the Lord.

1 Timothy 2:1 (NLT)

I urge you, first of all, to pray for all people. Ask God to help them; intercede on their behalf, and give thanks for them.

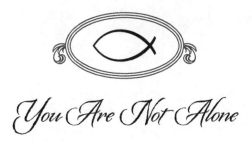

You Are Not Alone

SOMEONE IS PRAYING FOR YOU. I'M praying for you. It is very important to understand that you are not alone. There are saints all over the world that have lifted you up in prayer. They don't have to know you personally. They have been instructed as Christians to intercede for you through prayer. Many have been obedient and thus you have been lifted in prayer to the Almighty God.

You may feel alone, you may even have to go to appointments alone, stays at the hospital, alone. But you are on the mind and hearts of many. You will always need prayer. So do others. As you come to a point to know the true power of prayer and the command to pray for one another, you too will intercede on the behalf of others as they travel through the journey of cancer.

This journey is rough. No one likes to travel it alone. Knowing that someone, somewhere is praying for you makes the journey a little less rocky.

Obadiah 1:1(NLT)

*This is the vision that the Sovereign Lord revealed
to Obadiah concerning the land of Edom.
Edom's Judgment Announced We have heard a message from
the Lord that an ambassador was sent to the nations to say, "Get
ready, everyone! Let's assemble our armies and attack Edom!*

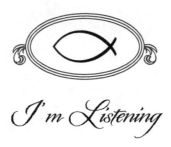

I'm Listening

WHAT HAVE YOU HEARD FROM THE Lord? Hearing from God takes a discerning ear and a relationship with God. God will speak to you in so many different ways. Be prepared and be open to the voice of God. God will speak to you through other people, through His word in the bible, through confirmation and in time. God may tell you to keep still. If so, that means His timing is very important to your next move. If God is telling you to make a move on a decision then stay in constant prayer to ensure you are staying in step with his direction.

Have you not heard the voice of God? Wait on God. God hears the prayers of his people. The bible teaches us in Matthew 6:26 to "look at the birds of the air; they do not sow or reap or store away in barns, and yet your heavenly Father feeds them. Are you not much more valuable than they?" You are more valuable and loved more than anything God has created.

God will speak to you. Be patient and know that an answer will come. Listen and be sure you are listening to God and not to other voices.

Hebrews 11:6 (NLT)

And it is impossible to please God without faith. Anyone who wants to come to him must believe that God exists and that he rewards those who sincerely seek him.

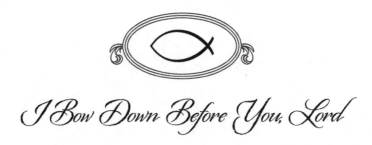

I Bow Down Before You, Lord

FAITH IS YOUR BIGGEST ALLY WHEN it comes to your healing and future. In order to have faith you first have to believe that God IS. You have to know that not only does He exists but that He is the ultimate power and only creator of life.

Coming before God is a humbling and powerful experience. For when you come to the Almighty you are experiencing an engagement that changes you from the inside out. This is your reward as you seek the Father with all your heart.

When God tells you something, He does not contradict Himself. You can be sure His promises are true.

Numbers 23:19 (NIV)

*God is not human, that he should lie, not a human
being, that he should change his mind. Does he speak and
then not act? Does he promise and not fulfill?*

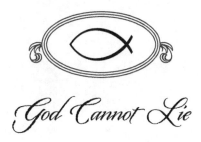

God Cannot Lie

PEOPLE LIE. PEOPLE EXAGGERATE. PEOPLE DO a lot of things that are not pleasing and acceptable to God.

Our God is not a man. He does not need to nor does He or would desire to lie to us. His promises are true. If God told you He would do something; He will. If you have claimed a promise from God, keep believing. The outward manifestations of those promises may not appear at the time you feel it is most needed. That is because your timing and God's timing are different. Your timing may come from desperation. His timing is divine, coming at a time that is perfect for your protection, purpose and destiny.

God's answers to your situation will not always look the way you envision it. Don't put God in a box. He'll never fit.

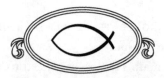

Nothing that you go through will be wasted.

Notes

_____

_____

_____

_____

_____

_____

_____

_____

_____

Notes

Notes

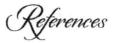

References

of the National Council of the Churches of Christ in the United States of America. Used by permission. All rights reserved.

Scripture quotations marked "MSG" or "The Message" are taken from The Message. Copyright 1993, 1994, 1995, 1996, 2000, 2001, 2002. Used by permission of NavPress Publishing Group.

Scripture Index

Romans 10:9 (NIV)

John 9:2 (NIV)

2 Peter 1:3 (NIV)

1 Thessalonians 1:2-5 (NLT)

Deuteronomy 4:29 (NLT)

Galatians 6:6:1-3 (NLT)

John 13:7 (NLT)

Psalm 25:16 (NLT)

Mark 11:24 (NLT)

Matthew 9:28-30 (NLT)

Revelation 20:10 (NLT)

Ephesians 6:13 (NLT)

1 Corinthians 2:9 (NLT)

I Peter 4:12-13 (ESV)

Daniel 8:27 (MSG)

Exodus 15:11 (NLT)

John 9:2 (TLB)

Job 5:19 (NLT)

James 1:2-3 (NLT)

Romans 8:18 (ESV)

Proverbs 21:31 (NLT)

Genesis 15:6 (NLT)

Jeremiah 30:17(NIV)

Lamentations 3:31-33(ESV)

Psalm 27:14 (NIV)

Romans 8:39 (NIV)

Jeremiah 17:14 (NIV)

John 16:33 (NIV)

Isaiah 30:21 (NIV)

2 Peter 3:9 (NLT)

Mark 11:22-23 (NIV)

Hebrews 10:23 (NIV)

James 5:14-15 (NIV)

Psalm 22:24 (NLT)

Proverbs 3:24 (NLT)

Ecclesiastes 3:1 (NLT)

1 Corinthians 2:9 (KJV)

1 Samuel 1:10 (NLT)

Micah 1:3 (NLT)

Galatians 3:28 (NLT)

Nahum 1:7 (NLT)

Matthew 17:19

Haggai 2:19 (NIV)

Matthew 6:34 (NIV)

Amos 3:3 (NLT)

2 Corinthians 1:4 (NLT)

Ruth 3:5 (NLT)

Joshua 5:5

1 Peter 3:3-4 (NLT)

2 Samuel 1:7 (NLT)

Job 22:28 (NIV)

Jonah 2:2 (NLT)

1 Kings 8:23 (NLT)

Hebrews 11:1

Daniel 2:3 (NLT)

Habakkuk 1:2 (NLT)

Jeremiah 29:11 (NIV)

Zephaniah 3:9 (NLT)

Psalm 94:19 (NRSV)

Prov. 16:33 (CEV)

2 Kings 5:10 (NLT)

Romans 12:4-5 (NIV)

Joel 2:7 (NLT)

Jeremiah 20:14-15 (KJV)

2 Corinthians 1:5 (NLT)

Romans 8:35-39 (NIV)

Psalm 77:11 (NIV)

2 Timothy 3:16 (NIV)

Romans 8:38-39 (NRSV)

I Chronicles 5:20 (NRSV)

1 Samuel 16:7 (NRSV)

Jeremiah 29:11(NRSV)

Proverbs 1:33 (NRSV)

Romans 10:9 (NRSV)

Romans 8:28(NIV)

Jeremiah 29:11(NIV)

Matthew 6:34 (NLT)

Mark 5:22-24 (NIV)

Deuteronomy 4:9 (NLT)

1 Thessalonians 5:18 (NLT)

Genesis 28:15 (NLT)

Romans 12:12 (NLT)

Joshua 24:15 (NIV)

Jeremiah 17:7 (NLT)

John 6:68 (NLT)

2 Thessalonians 1:3 (NLT)

John 13:17 (NLT)

John 14:27 (NIV)

Psalm 71:20 (NIV)

James 1:5-6 (NIV)

Psalm 138:7 (NIV)

Philippians 4:12-13 (NIV)

1 Samuel 3:10 (NIV)

1 Peter 1:21 (NLT)

Habakkuk 2:3 (NLT)

Titus 3:4-6 (NLT)

1 Chronicles 4:10 (NLT)

Zechariah 13:9 (NLT)

John 16:33

1 John 5:14-15 (NLT)

Galatians 2:20 (NLT)

Galatians 6:2 (NLT)

James 1:5 (NLT)

Nehemiah 9:6 (NLT)

Revelation 14:13 (NLT)

Hebrews 4:12 (NLT)

John 10:10 (NLT)

Ezra 10:12 (NLT)

Malachi 3:16-18 (MSG)

Song of Solomon 2:11 (NLT)

Leviticus 8:10-12 (NLT)

Jude 1:2 (NLT)

Luke 10:34 (NLT)

Mark 1:17 (NLT)

Ephesians 6:18-20 (MSG)

Ezekiel 37:14 (NLT)

Judges 6:23 (NIV)

2 Chronicles 9:6 (NLT)

2 John 1:12 (NLT)

Joel 2:21 (NLT)

Colossians 3:13 (NLT)

Esther 4:14 (NLT)

Acts 1:7 (NLT)

Nehemiah 1:4 (NLT)

Philemon 1:22 (NLT)

Lamentations 3:22 (NLT)

Hosea 6:2 (NIV)

3 John 1:4 (NLT)

Isaiah 40:31 (NLT)

1 Timothy 2:1 (NLT)

Obadiah 1:1(NLT)

Matthew 6:26 (NIV)

Hebrews 11:6 (NLT)

Numbers 23:19 (NIV)

Do You Want To Be Saved?

Romans 10:9 (NIV)

If you declare with your mouth, Jesus is Lord, and believe in your heart that God raised him from the dead, you will be saved.

You can ask Christ into your life right now. I will never assume that everyone reading this devotional has committed their life to Christ. If you would like to accept Christ into your life say and believe the following words, from your lips to Gods' ears.

> *"God, I have sinned and now I want to turn from my past and ask for your forgiveness. I believe that your son, Jesus Christ died for my sins, rose from the dead, is alive and hears this prayer. I want Jesus to become the Lord of my life, and reign in my heart from this day forward. I ask that you send the Holy Spirit to help me do your will for the rest of my life. In Jesus name I pray. Amen!*

That's it. If you believed this prayer you are now born again. This is just the beginning of your transformation. You are now His child and He's your God. Jesus Christ is now your Lord and savior. Please go to my website to help you with your next steps.

www.revcheryl.com

Visit Rev. Cheryl

Website
www.revcheryl.com

Instagram
RevCherylTaylor

Twitter
@revcheryltaylor

Facebook
Taylormade LLC *or* Rev Cheryl

CPSIA information can be obtained
at www.ICGtesting.com
Printed in the USA
LVHW112336030220
645691LV00003B/432